Peripheral Vascular Disease in Primary Care

This book is due for return on or before the last date shown below.

CHRONIC DISEASES IN PRIMARY CARE

Peripheral Vascular Disease in Primary Care

ANITA SHARMA
MBBS, MD, DRCOG, MFFP
General Practitioner
Oldham

Contributions by
JOANNE WHITMORE
and
ADELE MARIE SCIMONE

Forewords by

MICHAEL TAYLOR
General Practitioner
Heywood, Middleton and Rochdale PCT

DEEPAK BHATNAGAR
Consultant/Senior Lecturer in Diabetes and Metabolism
Royal Oldham Hospital
University of Manchester
Cardiovascular Research Group

and

GAIL RICHARDS
Chief Executive, NHS Oldham

Radcliffe Publishing
London • New York

Radcliffe Publishing Ltd
33–41 Dallington Street
London
EC1V 0BB
United Kingdom

www.radcliffepublishing.com

Electronic catalogue and worldwide online ordering facility.

British Library Cataloguing in Publication Data

A catalogue record for this book is available from the British Library.

ISBN-13: 978 184619 435 1

The paper used for the text pages of this book is FSC® certified. FSC (The Forest Stewardship Council®) is an international network to promote responsible management of the world's forests.

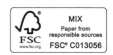

Typeset by Pindar NZ, Auckland, New Zealand
Printed and bound by TJI Digital, Padstow, Cornwall, UK

Contents

Foreword by Michael Taylor

Whether peripheral vascular disease is your passion or simply is recognised as an important component of your daily work, I have not the least hesitation in recommending this book to you. *Peripheral Vascular Disease in Primary Care* lays out in its chapters comprehensive information with the appropriate amount of detail to satisfy the most ardent general practitioner (GP) with a special interest in this subject. However, largely written and completely edited by a GP, Dr Anita Sharma, it has a style that is lean and sparse while nonetheless remaining a pleasure for any busy professional to read.

It is a book to relish rather than devour in that it lends itself to reading one or a few chapters at a time rather than cover to cover in a single sitting. It is therefore an excellent source and reference book for all primary care professionals. This attribute is enhanced by the fact that the author has had the opportunity to consult widely, including specialist colleagues, both doctors and nurses.

Having had the privilege and pleasure of contributing to the learning of students, nurses and registrars I am well aware of the suitability of this book for their purposes. They will be surprised with the descriptions of various pathologies simply explained, which they will seldom have noticed while working on hospital wards.

As it goes to press this book is completely up to date and is unlikely to need revision for many years. Chapter 15, on commissioning services for peripheral vascular disease, is particularly timely as the National Health Service enters a period of austerity and GP commissioning.

To summarise, this is a pragmatic book written by a GP and her team for GP teams; it should, therefore, find a place on the bookshelves of busy practices.

Dr Michael Taylor BSc, MB, ChB, MRCGP MICGP
General Practitioner
Heywood, Middleton and Rochdale PCT
January 2011

Foreword by Deepak Bhatnagar

Clinical professionals generally do not perceive the peripheral vasculature as an important site of disease as compared with the organs in the major cavities of the body. Neglected in this way, pathology in the peripheral vascular system often presents clinically in an advanced stage or in a dramatic, life-threatening manner. It is, therefore, important that symptoms and signs of disease are recognised early.

Peripheral vascular disease is thought to be more prevalent in the older age group, but it is important to appreciate that it can occur prematurely in certain high-risk groups such as people with diabetes or lipid disorders. As with most conditions lifestyle-related factors such as diet, smoking and obesity often play a major role in the causation of disease in the peripheral vasculature. This book offers the reader a very useful overview of peripheral vascular disease as well as suggesting models of care.

Those working in primary care need to be able to recognise not only the acute presentations of peripheral vascular disease – such as critical limb ischaemia or deep-vein thrombosis – but also manage the preventative aspects and routine treatment of conditions such as varicose veins, intermittent claudication, leg ulcers and the diabetic foot. If managed poorly peripheral vascular disease can lead to problems with tissue viability. The good news is that the framework for diagnosing and managing many of these conditions in the community is gradually being put in place. This should avoid unnecessary admissions to hospital, but it is important that any management strategy is integrated with secondary care so that the patient pathway is seamless, with easy and timely access to any level of care.

The shift to primary care management accompanied with guidelines from the National Institute for Health and Clinical Excellence is well presented in this book.

Dr Anita Sharma's book covers the essentials of conditions involving the arterial and venous system. It should be a welcome source of knowledge and information, particularly for those working in a primary care setting with the aim of improving their standards of care.

Dr Deepak Bhatnagar TD MBBS PhD FRCP FRCPI FRCPath FAHA
Consultant/Senior Lecturer in Diabetes and Metabolism
Royal Oldham Hospital and University of Manchester
Cardiovascular Research Group
January 2011

Foreword by Gail Richards

The role of primary care is unique in this country, bringing continuity of care and a wealth of understanding about patients' experiences and acting as the 'navigator' through our complex health and social care system.

General practitioners (GPs), pharmacists and all primary care staff are uniquely placed to make continual improvements across pathways of care, supporting their patients in a broad range of health conditions and circumstances. They are always eager to gain new, updated knowledge and information to help them achieve this.

This valuable book makes a significant contribution to the care of patients with peripheral vascular disease (PVD). It recognises our clear duty to provide effective education and support for patients, their families and carers. For PVD patients, we hope that our ability to improve their quality of life and manage pain effectively will continue to grow. Ensuring that all patients access the best treatment so that they can live longer and more fulfilled lives is always the primary care aim.

Anita Sharma is an experienced, practising GP whose book on PVD offers new insights for primary care professionals and is a generous contribution to the work of primary care practitioners everywhere.

Gail Richards
Chief Executive, NHS Oldham (2002–10)
January 2011

Preface

Peripheral vascular disease (PVD) is common and has a significant adverse effect on the quality of life. It is a marker of substantially increased cardiovascular risk. One in six people over the age of 55 years has peripheral arterial disease (PAD). A general practice with a list size of 6000 patients will have approximately 30 symptomatic patients with PVD. About 60% of patients with PVD have no symptoms, so screening high-risk patients is useful.

As PVD fails to make it into the Quality and Outcomes Framework – it seems that it has been overlooked and sometimes forgotten – the general practitioner (GP) has a vital role of coordinating vascular risk factor management in primary care.

Higher incidence is seen in smokers, diabetics and people with renal disease. Smoking is the single biggest risk factor for PAD. Effective management of PVD by providing a one-stop clinic in the community helps to prevent crises, deterioration and admission to expensive secondary care.

We are living in an era characterised by continual improvement in condition management, patient choice and economic constriction. The opportunity for treating PVD in the primary care closer to the patient's home should be explored by commissioning.

This book is a concise and practical guide to recognising, managing and reducing the cardiovascular risk factors in patients with PVD. Throughout this book I have tried to simplify the diagnosis and management, keeping it relevant to the busy GP. This book is intended as a means of refining the reader's knowledge in readiness for change and identifying areas in which further in-depth study is needed. This book enlightens not only GPs but also GPwSIs (general practitioners with a special interest), practice nurses, district nurses and nurses involved in vascular and diabetic clinics. The book also contains something of interest for medical students, foundation doctors and GP specialist registrars. There are references given at the end of each chapter for those who wish to learn more.

If you gain some expertise as a result of reading this book it will have served its purpose well.

Anita Sharma
January 2011

About the author

Anita Sharma MBBS, MD, DRCOG, MFFP has been a general practitioner in Oldham for more than 22 years and loves every second of working as a GP.

She is an undergraduate trainer attached to the University of Manchester and is a trainer in family planning. She is the GP editor for the *British Journal of Medical Practitioners* and *JuniorDr*, the magazine for trainee doctors. She writes regularly in various GP magazines on clinical and practice developmental issues.

Anita has served as a Local Medical Committee locality member for the last 7 years and is a GP appraiser for Oldham Primary Care Trust. She is also the chairperson of the Rochdale Division of the British Medical Association and organises various educational and social activities.

With the help and support of her patient participation group, she organises various fundraising activities and raises money for Cancer Research UK. She has donated the royalties raised by her recently published book *COPD in Primary Care* (2010), by Radcliffe Publishing, to Breathe Easy Oldham.

Contributors

Joanne Whitmore has worked as a nurse in cardiology for over 15 years in a variety of roles encompassing primary and secondary care. Shortly after qualifying at Bury General Hospital, Joanne worked on coronary care units at Bury and later at Oldham, where she also worked part time as a research nurse responsible for Phase 3 clinical trials.

After a brief spell in management, Joanne returned to cardiology, involved in acute chest pain management and thrombolysis. Following a secondment with Heywood, Middleton and Rochdale Primary Care Trust as a health improvement practitioner within the primary prevention team, Joanne was employed by NHS Oldham, where she currently works as the CHD Service Coordinator.

Her main interests include primary prevention, management of risk factors and the management of blood pressure in primary care. She is a member of the Primary Care Cardiovascular Society (PCCS), Cardiovascular Nurse Leaders, British Association for Nurses in Cardiac Care (BANCC) and the European Society of Cardiology (ESC) Council on Cardiovascular Nursing and Allied Professionals.

Adele Marie Scimone qualified as a registered nurse in 1997 and worked for 5 years in an orthopaedic trauma unit. This is where she developed a passion for wound care and prevention of pressure ulcers, working as Viability Link Nurse during this time.

She then took a post as Community Staff Nurse with Oldham Primary Care Trust in order to gain experience in leg ulcer management. This led to a secondment on the Community Specialist Practitioner degree programme where she gained a BSc (Hons). After carrying out the role of District Nurse in 2008 she obtained her current post of Clinical Nurse Specialist in Tissue Viability for Oldham Community Services, where she leads a small team. She is currently working towards her Masters degree.

Acknowledgements

Every piece of writing takes time – the time that could have been spent with my husband and two children.

My heartfelt gratitude goes to my husband, Ravi, a consultant physician, for his continued support and for doing my household duties while I battled with my computer.

I owe a considerable debt of gratitude to my two children: my son Neel, who is currently doing a MSc in Gastroenterology, and my daughter Ravnita, an anaesthetist in Manchester. They had to suffer weekends where I was present in shape and form in the household but absent from the family.

I am particularly grateful to Joanne Whitmore for her contribution towards aggressive management of patients with peripheral vascular disease to improve outcome and quality of life.

I would like to record my sincere thanks to Adele Marie Scimone for relating the principles of management of leg ulcers and use of correct grade of elastic support and dressing.

Successful management of diabetic foot requires the skills of not only the general practitioner but also the practice nurse. I am fortunate to have Kathryn Mkandawire, who contributed to the chapter of diabetic foot.

I am very grateful indeed to Mr Hadfield, consultant vascular surgeon in Oldham, for editing the chapter on varicose veins.

I am indebted to my practice staff for the smooth running of the practice that helped me to concentrate on writing this book. I particularly wish to thank my healthcare assistant Anthony Kyle, for his computer skills and helping me to insert the tables and graphs.

My thanks also go to the patients who have given consent for the use of the photographs as illustrations in this book.

Finally, I wish to thank Michael Hawkes, Editorial Assistant at Radcliffe Publishing, for his tolerance and support.

I sincerely hope that you, the reader, agree that this has been time well spent.

Anita Sharma

Varicose veins

Definition

There are many definitions: perhaps the most useful is that varicose veins are dilated, elongated or tortuous superficial veins, irrespective of size.

Prevalence

Varicose veins are one of the more commonly presenting conditions in general practice. The incidence is increasing because of an increase in obesity and sedentary lifestyle.[1] The overall reported prevalence varies: 25%–30% in women and 10%–20% in men is frequently quoted, although a recent study in Scotland found 32% in women and 40% in men. It is seldom life-threatening, but can cause much morbidity in younger age groups. Despite the lower prevalence rate, women consult their general practitioner more than men, because of cosmetic reasons. The prevalence rate increases with age, with 80% in people over the age of 60 years. The complication rates are much higher in older people.

Predisposing factors
- Family history.
- Pregnancy.
- Multiparity.
- Obesity.

- Age.
- Previous deep-vein thrombosis (DVT).
- Prolonged standing.
- Sedentary lifestyle.
- Pelvic tumour.
- Congenital abnormality of veins.
- Arteriovenous fistula.

Types

- *Truncal varices* – involve the main stem and/or tributaries of long or short saphenous veins. Subcutaneous, palpable and 4 mm or more in diameter.
- *Reticular varices* – lie deeper, not palpable and less than 4 mm in diameter.
- *Telangiectasia* – also known as thread veins or spider veins. They may appear during pregnancy, menopause, old age or puberty. Thread veins are usually 1 mm or less in diameter.

Varicose veins may also be classified as:
- *Primary varicose veins* – these are varicose veins of undetermined aetiology.
- *Secondary varicose veins* – these usually develop following, for example, DVT, or occasionally trauma caused by stab wound or surgery.

Venous system

The venous system of the leg comprises a superficial system and a deep system. The superficial system comprises the long saphenous vein (LSV) and the short saphenous vein (SSV). The LSV passes anterior to the medial malleolus at the ankle, then up the medial leg and thigh, joining the common femoral vein 2 cm below and lateral to the pubic tubercle at the sapheno-femoral junction. The SSV passes posterior to the lateral malleolus at the ankle, up the posterior calf and joins the popliteal vein at the sapheno-popliteal junction about 2 cm above the knee crease. The superficial and deep venous systems are connected at various levels by perforating veins. Valves in the superficial veins, deep veins and the perforating veins prevent backflow.

Aetiology and physiology

Heredity

There is a familial tendency in varicose veins. The exact defect and its inheritance pattern are unknown but it may be a defect in the vein wall collagen or elastin.

Hormonal

There is a definite female hormonal relationship. In particular, progesterone inhibits smooth muscle contraction in the vein wall and may allow the vein to dilate to the point of the valve giving way.

Muscular compartment forces

The pumping action of the muscles of the calf and the foot, aided by the respiratory movements of the diaphragm, compresses the veins. One-way valves prevent reflux from the deep system to the superficial system. Compartment pressures can reach and exceed 150 mmHg; this can cause sudden 'giving-way' of the valves and the subsequent development of varicose veins.

Hydrostatic forces

These are due to the weight of the blood column from heart down to the affected vein in the leg and can be seen to contribute to progressively more distal venous incompetence. The weakness of the vein valve leads to dilatation and separation of valve cusps, resulting in incompetence. Blood flows from the deep to the superficial veins, causing further dilatation.

Symptoms

- Cosmetic disfigurement (the most commonly presenting symptom).
- Aching/throbbing legs.
- Tiredness.
- Heavy feeling.
- Leg swelling.
- Itching.
- Restless legs.
- Nocturnal cramps.

The pain or aching is worse after prolonged standing or towards the end of the day and may be relieved by leg elevation and support stockings. Symptoms may be worse in hot weather or in premenstrual women.

Pregnant women are more likely to develop varicose veins due to the mechanical pressure of an enlarged uterus over the pelvic veins. The increasing concentration of progestogens, increased blood volume and increased pelvic blood flow cause relaxation and dilatation of the vein walls. Most women see an improvement in their varicose veins after the pregnancy is over.

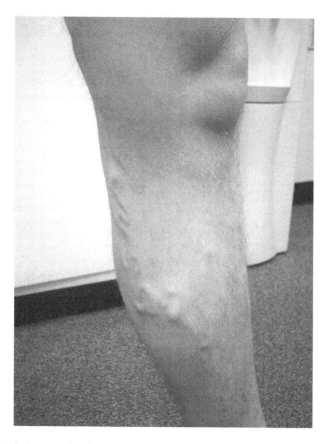

FIGURE 1.1 Varicose veins leg

Causes of leg swelling

- DVT.
- Superficial thrombophlebitis.
- Gravitational oedema.
- Lymphoedema.
- Lipoedema.
- Renal causes.
- Hypoproteinemia.
- Liver disease.
- Thyroid problem.

Examination

The patient should be examined standing up in a warm room.

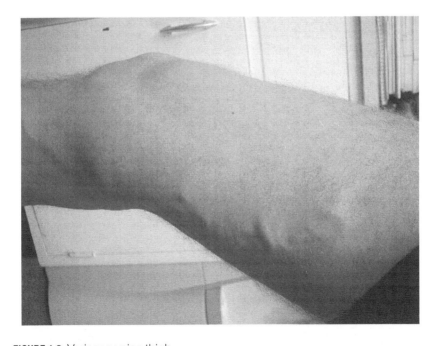

FIGURE 1.2 Varicose veins thigh

Inspection

Look for the following:

- oedema
- eczema
- ulcer
- lipodermatosclerosis
- distribution of veins (long saphenous distribution is thigh and medial side of calf; short saphenous distribution is below the knee on the lateral and posterior side of calf).

Palpation

Abdominal and pelvic examination must be done to exclude secondary causes. Percussion over the varices may help trace their course.

Trendelenburg test

This is to determine the site of incompetence. However, it is increasingly of historic significance only, as the use of handheld Dopplers has supplanted it. Ask the patient to lie down. Elevate the leg and apply a tourniquet below the sapheno-femoral junction. Now ask the patient to stand up. If the varicosities do not fill up, but fill on release of pressure, the incompetence at the sapheno-femoral junction is confirmed. The use of a handheld Doppler to insonate over the sites of incompetence and demonstrate reflux is now considered an essential part of the examination.

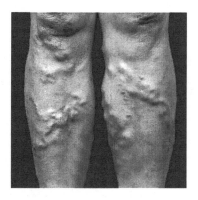

FIGURE 1.3 Varicose veins examination

Investigations

- Height, weight and body mass index.
- Blood pressure check.
- Full blood count, serum ferritin, serum B_{12} and folate level, kidney function tests (U&E), thyroid function test (TFT), and liver function test (LFT).
- Routine urine check for protein, sugar.
- Doppler (as above).
- Duplex scanning.

Duplex scanning can accurately assess the venous incompetence and map the pattern of varicose veins. Ideally it would be used in all patients for whom treatment is being considered. At the very least it should be used for all recurrent varicose veins, for patients with short saphenous incompetence and for patients with complications.

Management[1]

Many patients require:
- Reassurance
- Education regarding weight reduction
- Dietary advice. Low fat (cholesterol), high fibre diet incorporating fresh fruit and vegetables (in line with published cardioprotective dietary advice)
- Exercise advice
- Simple advice regarding – avoiding standing for long period of time and leg elevation when sitting down
- Support stockings if symptoms are troublesome. These can be issued on FP10.

In the last decade there have been major changes in the management of varicose veins. Sometimes a patient may need more than one type of treatment to achieve a good outcome. Each procedure has its own limitations and complications and these should be explained to the patient. The treatment options are:
- compression hosiery
- sclerotherapy

- surgical intervention
- endovenous laser ablation
- radiofrequency ablation.

Compression hosiery

Compression hosiery has no long-term benefit in preventing the progression of varicose veins or recurrence after treatment and it is only effective as long as the patient wears it. Class 2 stocking has a pressure range of 18–24 mm of mercury. It can improve the symptom control in patients with uncomplicated varicose veins. Poor patient compliance is the main drawback, with reports suggesting a compliance of 37%–39%.[2,3] If stockings are badly worn they can cause necrosis of the skin, especially in diabetics with impaired sensation. If the Ankle Brachial Pressure Index is less than 0.9 then compression hosiery should be avoided.

Sclerotherapy

Sclerotherapy is a common treatment. Currently used sclerosants are sodium tetradecyl sulfate 0.5%–3% or polidocanol 0.5%–3%. Foam is prepared using one part of sclerosant mixed with four parts of air. A venflon is sited in the vein before injecting the foam. The leg is elevated to empty the vein. A maximum of 12 mL of foam is used in one session. Compression hosiery is applied for 1–2 weeks.

Sclerotherapy is suitable for telangiectasia, small veins in the absence of axial or junctional reflux or residual varicosities following surgical treatment. Patients are advised not to drive for 30 minutes afterward sclerotherapy as visual disturbance may occur (in less than 2% of cases) but resolves within 30 minutes. DVT is rare – less than 2%.

This treatment may be carried out on an outpatient basis but should be done by a practitioner trained in the technique. There is a very small risk of anaphylaxis so resuscitation equipment must be available.

Ultrasound-guided foam sclerotherapy is a minimally invasive alternative to conventional surgery. A questionnaire-based survey of patients who had foam sclerotherapy and those who underwent conventional surgery showed that those who had foam treatment had less pain, reduced analgesia, less time off work and were quicker to return to driving.[4] Patients who had surgery were more likely to have significant bruising and pain.[3]

Surgical intervention

DVT risk assessment should be done in patients undergoing varicose vein surgery. All high-risk patients should receive prophylactic treatment as per National Institute for Health and Clinical Excellence (NICE) guidelines. Standard varicose vein surgery is still the most common surgical intervention.

Great saphenous vein (GSV) surgery involves ligation of the sapheno-femoral junction, division of tributaries and stripping of great saphenous vein up to the level of knee.

Short saphenous vein (SSV) surgery involves ligation of the sapheno-popliteal junction and multiple stab avulsions.

Ligation of sapheno-femoral or sapheno-popliteal junction with stripping of the long saphenous vein and multiple avulsion of varicosities is done either under general anaesthetic or epidural. The results of short saphenous vein (SSV) surgery are not as good as great saphenous vein (GSV) surgery. There is persistent reflux in up to 25% of cases.[5] On the whole this will be carried out as a day-case procedure. Post-operatively the patient wears compression hosiery for 1–2 weeks and is encouraged to mobilise back to normal activity as soon as possible. The patient is warned to expect quite extensive bruising and palpable subcutaneous lumpiness along the track of the vein. Time taken to return to full activity varies but an average of 1–2 weeks is the norm. No hospital follow-up is usually required, unless further treatment is already planned.

Endovenous laser ablation (EVLA)

The procedure should be undertaken according to current NICE guidelines. The vein is canulated using duplex ultrasound. A laser fibre is inserted in to the incompetent vein. Endovenous ablation was initially used for great saphenous vein reflux only. It has been shown to be successful in small saphenous vein reflux.

Post-treatment discomfort, thermal injury, cutaneous nerve injury, DVT and hyperpigmentation are some, albeit rare, complications.

Radiofrequency ablation (RFA)

Intervention should be undertaken according to the current NICE guidelines. The vein is canulated under duplex ultrasound control. Radiofrequency ablation uses a bipolar endovenous catheter that generates a temperature of 85–120 degree centigrade at the vein wall. The radiofrequency ablation probe should be sited 2 cm below to the sapheno-femoral junction or sapheno-popliteal junction. VNUS ClosureFAST technique allows 7 cm segments to be treated in 20 seconds. VNUS Closure Fast system has been reported to have an occlusion rate of 99.6% at two years in the hands of experts. Nerve damage, skin burns and deep-vein thrombosis are some rare complications.

When to refer: NICE referral guidelines for varicose veins[6]

Immediate

- Bleeding from a varicosity that has eroded the skin.

Urgent

- A varicosity that has bled and is at a risk of another bleed.

Soon

- An ulcer that is painful and progressive, despite treatment.

Routine

- Active or healed ulcer and/or progressive changes that may benefit from surgery.
- Troublesome symptoms and the general practitioner and/or the patient feels the varicosities are having a severe impact on the quality of life.
- Recurrent superficial thrombophlebitis.

KEY POINTS
- Obesity, previous DVT and prolonged standing are the main predisposing factors.
- Reassurance, education and advice about weight management, exercise and support hosiery is all that is needed in the majority of patients.
- Ultrasound-guided foam sclerotherapy and endovenous laser ablation are minimally invasive alternatives to conventional surgery.
- The National Institute for Health and Clinical Excellence has recommended which patients should be referred for specialist assessment (NICE guidelines).

Further reading

- Varicose veins, article available at: www.emedicine.com/med/topic2788.htm.
- Site with some pictures from an American surgical perspective: www.vascular. co.nz/varicose_vein_links.htm.

References

1 Campbell B. Varicose veins and their management. *BMJ*. 2006; **333**(7562): 287–92.

2 Chant ADB, Davies IJ, Pike JM *et al*. Support stockings in practical management of varicose veins. *Phlebology*. 1989; **4**: 167–9.

3 Raju S, Hollis K, Neglen P. Use of compression stockings in chronic venous disease: patient compliance and efficacy. *Ann Vasc Surg*. 2007; **21**(6): 790–5.

4 Darvall KAL, Bate GR, Adam DJ *et al*. Recovery after ultrasound-guided foam sclerotherapy compared with conventional surgery for varicose veins. *Br J Surg*. 2009; **96**(11): 1262–7.

5 Rashid HI, Ajeel A, Tyrrell MR. Persistent popliteal fossa reflux following saphenopopliteal disconnection. *Br J Surg*. 2002; **89**(6): 748–51.

6 National Institute for Health and Clinical Excellence. *Varicose Veins*. 2001/043 NICE issues advice on appropriate referral from general practitioner. www.nice.org.uk/newsroom/pressreleases/pressreleasearchive/press releases2001/2001_043__nice_issues_advice_on_appropriate_referral_from_ general_to_specialist_services.jsp (accessed 10 March 2011).

2

Deep-vein thrombosis

Incidence

The incidence of deep-vein thrombosis (DVT) among younger people is two to three per 10 000 per annum[1]; much lower than the older population, which is estimated at 20 per 10 000 per annum,[1] a probable underestimate as asymptomatic patients are not included.

Risk

Patients with the following factors are at risk of developing DVT:
- old age
- malignancy
- immobility
- obesity (body mass index over 30 kg/m^2)
- dehydration
- recent surgery
- acute medical illness
- previous history of DVT
- varicose veins with phlebitis
- first-degree relative with a history of venous thromboembolism (VTE)
- certain inherited conditions such as Factor V Leiden thrombophilia (this increases the blood's tendency to clot)
- thrombocytopenia

- polycythaemia
- puerperium
- hormone replacement therapy or combined contraceptive pill
- pregnancy.

There is an estimated 25 000 deaths each year due to hospital-acquired venous thromboembolism (VTE) – deep-vein thrombosis and the potentially fatal pulmonary embolism and many of these are preventable. Despite the evidence for the benefits of thromboprophylaxis, this is only used in half of eligible patients and many professionals are not aware of the risk of VTE.

Patients with either occult cancer or clinically diagnosed cancer are at increased risk of thromboembolism. The largest prospective study of acute VTE – RIETE, the Computerized Registry of Patients with Venous Thromboembolism – has more than 17 000 patients.[2] Occult cancer was detected in 1.2% of the patients and 16% had cancer diagnosed before thromboembolism or during admission.

Signs and symptoms

- Some 80% of DVTs are asymptomatic.
- Leg pain.
- Warmth.
- Swelling.

Diagnosis

The diagnosis of DVT remains a challenge because of non-specific signs and symptoms. Both under-diagnosis and over-diagnosis can result in significant morbidity and mortality.

Assessment

A suspected DVT patient should have the risk assessment done using the Wells Risk Probability Scoring System. The scoring system takes into account the patient's history, clinical findings and possible alternative diagnosis. The scoring system is a tool for assessing the pretest probability of a DVT. A past history of DVT is the single strongest risk factor of a recurrent DVT.

TABLE 2.1 Wells Risk Probability Scoring System[3]

HISTORY	SCORE
Paralysis/paresis or plaster immobilisation of lower limb(s).	+1
Major surgery in past 4 weeks, or being bedridden for 3 or more days, or travel lasting longer than 4 hours in the previous 6 weeks.	+1
Cancer treatment in the previous 6 weeks or on palliative treatment.	+1
CLINICAL FINDINGS	**SCORE**
Entire leg swollen.	+1
Calf swollen, in the symptomatic leg the circumference is 3 cm more than the other leg, measured 10 cm below the tibial tuberosity.	+1
Tenderness along deep veins.	+1
Pitting oedema (worse in the symptomatic leg).	+1
Collateral superficial veins (non-varicose).	+1
POSSIBLE ALTERNATIVE DIAGNOSIS	**SCORE**
Musculoskeletal injuries, chronic oedema, superficial phlebitis in varicose veins of the leg, cellulitis of the leg, arthritis of the leg, Baker's cyst, haematoma.	−2

Total score	0 or less	1–2	3 or more
Risk of DVT	3% (low)	17% (mod)	75% (high)

Use Read codes:
- 388z – Wells DVT clinical probability score
- 140b0 – low probability
- 140b1 – moderate probability
- 140b2 – high probability.

D-dimers

D-dimers are fibrin degradation products and result from endogenous fibrinolysis associated with thrombus formation. The D-dimer test is best used in conjunction with the Wells Risk Probability Scoring System. A positive D-dimer indicates that VTE is a possibility and imaging of the legs should be the next step. However, false elevation of D-dimer can occur in patients with malignancy, infection, infarction, pregnancy and those who have recently had surgery. If a D-dimer is negative in a patient with a low risk (Wells Risk Probability Score[3]) the chance of missing a VTE is less than 1%. The patient can be reassured and there is no need to proceed to further imaging.[4]

Timing of D-dimer assay may be relevant too. D-dimer falls a few weeks after thrombus formation. Immunosorbent assay D-dimer tests take a long time to do and, hence, are not useful in acute care. Second-generation assays provide results within an hour and point-of-care tests produce results within 10–15 minutes. The upper limit for normal D-dimer range should be higher in older people in whom multiple co-morbidities are common.[5] In one study, specificity of D-dimer in patients with suspected pulmonary embolism over the age of 80 was only 10%, compared with those under 40 years, where the specificity was 67%.[5]

Imaging

Ultrasound is cheaper and more convenient than venography and can be performed irrespective of renal function.[6] Ultrasound uses sound waves to create pictures of blood flowing through the arteries and veins of the affected leg. A special type of ultrasound – Doppler ultrasound – is used to find out the flow of blood through a blood vessel. Ultrasound is sensitive for proximal DVT but not for distal DVT.

Venography is performed if ultrasound does not provide a clear diagnosis. Dye is injected into a vein that makes a vein visible on the X-ray. Slow blood flow in the X-ray may indicate a blood clot. Venography should be used in patients with a past history of DVT, as ultrasound is unreliable.

Lung ventilation perfusion scan (V/Q scan)

This is done if there is suspicion of pulmonary embolism.

A single test

One way to confirm a suspected DVT is a single compression ultrasound of the whole leg. Researchers looked into the cases of 4731 patients who were not treated with anticoagulants after a single negative test. Thirty-four patients developed DVT over the next 3 months (0.7%). The overall risk of DVT after a negative test result was 0.57%. The researchers think it is low and whole-leg ultrasound needs further study.[7]

Differential diagnosis

- Cellulitis.
- Muscle strain.
- Ruptured Baker's cyst.
- Lymphangitis.
- Venous insufficiency.

Referral to hospital

Immediate referral

- Patient is pregnant and has a suspected DVT.
- Suspected pulmonary embolism.
- Bilateral DVT.
- Extension of DVT to the inferior vena cava.

Urgent referral

- Wells Risk Probability Score of 1 or more (see above).

An earlier appointment within 24 hours

- DVT suspected, even if the patient has a Wells Risk Probability Score of 0 or less (low-risk).

Treatment

The main aims of treatment are:
- stopping the clot getting bigger
- prevention of recurrence of DVT
- prevention of pulmonary embolism.

Anticoagulation

The cornerstone of the treatment of DVT has been intravenous unfractionated heparin. Long-term management in the United Kingdom has been oral warfarin – an oral vitamin K antagonist. Anticoagulation initially with heparin and then an oral warfarin is initiated as soon as the diagnosis is confirmed. Warfarin has a very narrow therapeutic range and requires regular blood tests to measure INR (international normalised ratio). The National Patient Safety Agency (NPSA) anticoagulant alert in 2007 highlighted the many potential risks of warfarin prescribing and introduced a multidisciplinary strategy to reduce risks.[8] The NPSA recommends at least annual assessment of patients who are on long-term warfarin.

INR monitoring is mostly provided by the hospital clinic, but recently, with the introduction of practice-based commissioning, some GPwSI (general practitioners with a special interest) provide this service in the primary care. The INR result determines the dose of warfarin so that the patient can be maintained within the therapeutic range. Approximately 1%–2% of patients suffer side effects due to bleeding and thromboembolic side effects.

Current guidelines suggest full-dose anticoagulant with a low-molecular-weight heparin (LMWH) while waiting for the results of imaging. Anticoagulation can be stopped if the imaging is negative. If a Doppler ultrasound shows a thrombus, warfarin should be started and LMWH stopped when the INR is greater than 2.

LMWH is more effective than unfractionated heparin; it is safer and has a lower rate of major bleeding.[9] All patients should have full blood count, clotting profile and renal function tests prior to starting the therapy. There is a risk of thrombocytopenia in 0.2%–5% of cases treated with LMWH.

Fondaparinux, a new therapeutic class of factor Xa inhibitors, binds to antithrombin specifically.[10] It is a once-daily subcutaneous injection of a fixed dose and requires no monitoring. The only contraindication is renal failure. It is licensed for the treatment of DVT, pulmonary embolism and prophylaxis of VTE.

The majority of patients can be treated at home. This is safe, cost-effective and well liked by patients.[11] The patients should know whom to contact in case of any problem.[11]

Oral anticoagulation with warfarin (or alternative if warfarin allergy) should be given for 6 months in patients with DVT and longer in those patients with risk factors.[12,14] Compared with warfarin, long-term treatment with LMWH may be preferable in patients with cancer.

New oral anticoagulants

Two new oral anticoagulants were licensed in 2008: Pradaxa (dabigatran) and Xarelto (rivaroxaban). They both are taken orally at a fixed dose daily and do not require regular blood monitoring. There are no significant side effects and no drug interactions. They are licensed for high-risk hip and knee replacement surgery. In due course these agents will be used in other high-risk surgical procedures.

Vena cava filters

A vena cava filter is used if a patient develops a blood clot while taking anti-coagulant or is intolerant / has contraindications to anticoagulants.

A filter is inserted in the vena cava. This catches the blood clot that breaks off in a vein, preventing pulmonary embolism.[13] A filter will not prevent a new blood clot from forming.

Graduated compression hosiery

Stockings are worn on the leg from the arch of the foot to just below or just above the knee. They can reduce the swelling that can occur after a DVT. The stockings are tighter at the ankle and become looser as they go up. This creates pressure, which prevents clotting. There are three types of pressure stockings:

- *support pantyhose* – they offer the least amount of pressure
- *over-the-counter compression hose* – these stockings provide a little more pressure than support pantyhose and can be bought from pharmacy stores
- *prescription-strength compression hose* – these offer the greatest amount of pressure and need to be fitted by a trained professional.

Patients should be advised not to buy stockings over the counter as they could be of the wrong size and can cause more harm.

The patient should undergo an assessment and accurate measurement by a professional before a compression stocking for use following a DVT is fitted. Stockings should be changed every 3–6 months.

Reducing post-thrombotic complication

Compression stockings, if used within 1 month of a DVT and continued for at least 1 year (ideally 2 years), reduce post-thrombotic syndrome.[13] The patient should be advised to wear stockings each day, putting them on when lying in bed before getting out of bed and wearing them for the whole day until going to bed. Older patients may find it difficult to wear stockings. Furthermore, older people may have poor circulation due to diabetes or poor mobility and this can cause more harm.

Prophylaxis

The National Institute for Health and Clinical Excellence (NICE, also NIHCE) guidance on the prevention of DVT in patients undergoing elective orthopaedic surgery recommends prophylaxis with a LMWH such as Clexane (enoxaparin) or the indirect factor Xa inhibitor fondaparinux (Arixtra) for 4 weeks after surgery.[15] However, many patients do not receive the recommended prophylaxis. One possible reason could be that patients are discharged from the hospital and are not taught the correct use of prophylaxis at home.

Oral prophylaxis

A new orally active antithrombotic agent licensed for VTE prophylaxis following knee and hip surgery is dabigatran. It is available as 75 mg and 110 mg capsules and prophylaxis should be provided for up to 4 weeks after the surgery. This saves the need for continuing subcutaneous injection after the discharge from hospital.

Statins

A study published in 2009 reported that statins may reduce the chances of healthy people getting a DVT. In this study the researchers looked at the drug rosuvastatin.[16] However, in this study, even though the participants were healthy, compared with the general population they were all at higher risk of developing cardiovascular risks. So, more research is needed before statins can be widely used to prevent DVT.

Prognosis

The immediate and long-term prognoses could be:
- pulmonary embolism
- recurrence of VTE

- post-thrombotic syndrome (there is an increased chance of post-thrombotic syndrome if a DVT develops in the thigh vein or if a patient is obese – recurrence of a DVT is associated with a sixfold increase in post-thrombotic syndrome)[17]
- death.

Preventing a deep-vein thrombosis

The following things may prevent a first or recurrent DVT:
- avoiding long periods of immobility such as sitting for long hours
- regular exercise of calf muscles.

Air travel and DVT

VTE after air travel was first recorded in 1954.[18,19] The annual risk of VTE is increased by 12% if one long-haul flight is taken yearly.[20] The average risk of death from flight-related VTE is small when compared with risk of death from injuries at work and in motor vehicle crashes.[20]

The risk of VTE is increased for only 2 weeks after a long-haul flight. Airlines should continue to advise passengers on how to minimise the risk.

Any individual at risk of VTE should be advised to have more soft drinks than alcohol while flying to prevent dehydration. They should be advised to walk around the plane. Well-fitting compression stockings are also of benefit. Patients with post-phlebitic syndrome should wear grade 2 compression stockings.

There is no evidence that taking low-dose aspirin reduces the risk of thrombosis. Because of the risk of gastric side effects it is not recommended.[21] High-risk patients can take a single dose of LMWH subcutaneously – dalteparin, 5000 units or tinzaparin, 3500 units – just prior to the departure.

Reducing the risk of DVT in patients admitted to hospital

General practitioners must advise patients to stop taking oestrogen-containing oral contraceptive or hormone replacement therapy 4 weeks before planned surgery. An alternative contraceptive advice must be given to those who stop taking the pill.

Patients discharged with anti-embolism stockings must be given advice regarding the benefits of wearing them, if not given at the time of discharge. District nursing help should be provided to those who are unable to remove and replace the stockings themselves.

At-risk patients admitted for surgery must be advised regarding the risk assessment on admission to determine their risk of developing a VTE.

e-Learning on venous thromboembolism

An e-learning programme, e-VTE, aims to raise awareness of VTE prevention in the hospital setting and explores the challenges faced by a primary care physician. This has been developed by the Chief Medical Officer's VTE Implementation Working Group in partnership with e-Learning for Healthcare.

The programme has a pre-learning questionnaire and post-learning assessment. The four sessions cover:
- demographics, epidemiology and the risks of VTE
- methods of thromboprophylaxis
- implementation of thromboprophylaxis in the hospital setting
- implementation of thromboprophylaxis in primary care.

Each session takes around 20 minutes to complete and at the end of each session a certificate can be obtained by entering your name, role, location and deanery (if appropriate) at the end of the questionnaire. This can be a part of personal development planning (PDP) and can be used for appraisal and revalidation.

KEY POINTS
- DVT is a potentially preventable problem with increased incidence in older population.
- Patients most at risk of DVT are those who have had a previous thrombosis, recent surgery or malignancy.
- The Wells scoring system is useful to predict a clinical diagnosis of DVT.
- Negative D-dimer rules out thromboembolism. Patients with a positive test should have imaging.

Further reading

- The Prevention of Venous Thromboembolism in Hospitalised Patients www.publications.parliament.uk/pa/cm200405/cmselect/.../99.pdf (accessed 10 March 2011).
- Department of Health Chief Medical Officer (2007). *Report of the Independent Expert Working Group on the Prevention of Venous Thromboembolism in Hospitalized Patients.* www.dh.gov.uk/en/Publicationsandstatistics/Publications/PublicationsPolicyAndGuidance/DH_073944 (accessed 10 March 2011).
- National Institute for Health and Clinical Excellence. *Venous Thromboembolism: reducing the risk: NICE Guideline 92.* London: NICE; 2010 www.nice.org.uk/guidance/CG92 (accessed 10 March 2011).

References

1 Fowkes FJ, Price JF, Fowkes FG. Incidence of diagnosed deep vein thrombosis in the general population: systematic review. *Eur J Vasc Endovasc Surg.* 2003; **25**(1): 1–5.

2 Trujillo-Santos J, Prandoni P, Rivron-Guillot K *et al.* Clinical outcome in patients with venous thromboembolism and hidden cancer: findings from the RIETE Registry. *J Thromb Haemost.* 2008; **6**(2): 251–5.

3 Wells PS, Anderson DR, Bormanis J *et al.* Value of assessment of pretest probability of deep-vein thrombosis in clinical management. *Lancet.* 1997; **350**(9094): 1795–8.

4 Kelly J, Hunt BJ. The utility of pretest probability assessment in patients with clinically suspected venous thromboembolism. *J Thromb Haemost.* 2003; **1**(9): 1888–96.

5 Righini M, Goehring C, Bounameaux H *et al.* Effect of age on the performance of common diagnostic tests for pulmonary embolism. *Am J Med.* 2000; **109**(5): 357–61.

6 Blann AD, Lip GY. Clinical review: venous thromboembolism. *BMJ.* 2006; **332**(7537): 364.

7 Scott M, Stevens, Murray *et al.* Single Ultrasound test may suffice to rule out DVT-critical care *Am J Med.* 2010; 123: 158–65.

8 National Patient Safety Agency. *Anticoagulant alert-Patient Safety Alert: actions that can make anticoagulant therapy safer.* March 2007. Available at: www.npsa.nhs.uk/EasySiteWeb/GatewayLink.aspx?alld=10797 (accessed 10 March 2011).

9 van Dongen CJ, van den Belt AGM, Prins MH *et al.* Fixed dose subcutaneous low molecular weight haparins versus adjusted dose unfractionated heparin for venous thromboembolism. *Cochrane Database Syst Rev.* 2001; (4): CD001100.

10 Bauer KA. New anticoagulants. *Hematology Am Soc Hematol Educ Program.* 2006; 450–6.

11 Othieno R, Abu Affan M, Okpo E. Home versus in-patient treatment for deep vein thrombosis. *Cochrane Database Syst Rev.* 2001, (2): CD003076.

12 Winter M, Keeling D, Sharpen F *et al.* Procedures for the outpatient management of patients with deep venous thrombosis. *Clin Lab Haematol.* 2005; **27**(1): 61–6.

13 Young T, Aukes J, Hughes R *et al.* Vena caval filters for the prevention of pulmonary embolism. *Cochrane Database Syst Rev.* 2007; (3): CD006212.

14 Snow V, Qaseem A, Barry P *et al.* Management of venous thromboembolism: a clinical practice guideline from the American College of Physicians and the American Academy of Family Physicians. *Ann Fam Med.* 2007: **5**(1); 74–80.

15 National Institute for Health and Clinical Excellence. *Venous Thromboembolism: reducing the risk: NICE Guideline 92.* London: NICE; 2010 www.nice.org.uk/guidance/CG92 (accessed 10 March 2011).

16 Glynn RJ, Danielson E, Fonseca FA *et al.* A randomized trial of rosuvastatin in the prevention of venous thromboembolism. *N Engl J Med.* 2009; **360**(18): 1851–61. Epub March 2009 (abstract).

17 Prandoni P, Lensing AWA, Cogo A *et al.* The long-term clinical course of acute deep venous thrombosis. *Ann Intern Med.* 1996; **125**(1): 1–7.

18 Homans J. Thrombosis of the leg veins due to prolonged sitting. *N Engl J Med.* 1954; **250**(4): 148–9.

19 Ansell JE. Air travel and venous thromboembolism: is the evidence in? *N Engl J Med.* 2001; **345**(11): 828–9.

20 Kelman CW, Kortt MA, Becker NG *et al.* Deep vein thrombosis and air travel: record linkage study. *BMJ.* 2003; **327**(7423): 1072.

21 Watson HG. Travel and thrombosis. *Blood Rev.* 2005; **19**(5): 235–41.

3

Oral contraceptives and deep-vein thrombosis

In the United Kingdom, of the 75% of women aged 16–49 years who are using some form of contraception 16% are using the combined oral contraceptive pill.[1] The combined oral contraceptive pill carries a small but real risk of venous thromboembolism (VTE). The incidence of VTE in healthy non-pregnant women not taking any contraceptive pill is around five per 110 000 per year. The risk of VTE during pregnancy is much higher: 60 per 100 000 woman-years.[9]

Studies published in 1995 suggested that oestrogen-dominant pills are associated with a higher risk of VTE. Oestrogens reduce the antithrombin III level and reduce platelet function, thus promoting intravascular coagulation. Oestrogens may also promote arterial thrombosis if there is existing arterial wall disease. Data from EURAS (the European Active Surveillance Study) suggested that there was no difference in VTE rates between any of the combined oral contraceptive pills studied, with an approximate incidence of 90 per 100 000 woman-years.[3]

Some epidemiological studies reported a greater risk in women taking third-generation combined oral contraceptive pills that contain progestogens like desogestrel (DSG) or gestodene (GSD) rather than those containing the progestogens levonorgestrel (LNG) or norethisterone (NET) – the so-called second-generation contraceptive pills.[4]

It is well known that LNG opposes the oestrogen-mediated rise in sex-hormone binding globulin and high-density lipoprotein cholesterol and even lowers it if enough is given.[3] However, any beneficial effect of LNG and NET on VTE risk may not be as great as epidemiology of 1995–96 data suggested. The incidence of VTE in women taking the third-generation contraceptive pills is about 25 per 100 000 woman-years compared with 15 per 100 000 woman-years taking the second-generation contraceptive pills.[4]

The advice in a press release from the Department of Health *found no safety concerns about third-generation desogestrel or gestodene progestogens.*[2] There is only a 1–2 per million difference in annual VTE mortality between the third-generation (DSG, GSD) and the second-generation (LNG, NET) pills.[4]

A body mass index (BMI) over 30 is a significant risk factor for VTE in women on the combined contraceptive pill. A BMI $> 30 \, \text{kg/m}^2$ carries a twofold risk of VTE. For women with a BMI of $35–39 \, \text{kg/m}^2$, the risks of using a combined contraceptive pill generally outweigh the benefits; for those with a BMI $> 40 \, \text{kg/m}^2$ the combined contraceptive pill carries an unacceptable health risk.[5]

VTE risks are much higher in women who are carriers of hereditary thrombotic conditions.[6,7] A thrombophilia screening is necessary if a patient's close relative has had a VTE under the age of 45 years without any other risk factors.

Smoking, diabetes and high blood pressure also increase the risks of thromboembolism.[6,8]

Two studies on the use of oral contraceptives and venous thromboembolism have been published recently and both found an increased risk of VTE with the third-generation combined oral contraceptives containing desogestrel, gestodene, cyproterone acetate and drospirenone rather than levonorgestrel. In the first example – the MEGA case-control study – cases were identified from the anticoagulant clinics in the Netherlands.[9] The second example is a retrospective study using information from the Danish registries.[10]

Arterial thromboembolism
The risk of myocardial infarction is not increased in healthy pill users compared with non-users. Smoking, high blood pressure, age, obesity and diabetes are additional risk factors in pill users. Women with risk factors for arterial disease have a significant increased risk of myocardial infarction if taking progesterone-dominant pills.[11]

It seems that although oestrogen-dominant pills increase the risk of VTE they may have some protection against atherosclerosis, compared with progestogen-dominant pills.[12]

Surgery and oral contraceptives

Oestrogenic contraceptive pills should be stopped 4 weeks before elective surgery. The National Institute for Health and Clinical Excellence (NICE, also NIHCE) concludes on oral contraception: 'If the decision to stop oral contraception is taken it is important that women are provided with advice on the use of contraceptives in the interim period'.[13] Contraceptive pills containing only progestogens need not be stopped before surgery. NICE does not include any advice on restarting the combined contraceptive pill after surgery, but the Faculty of Sexual and Reproductive Healthcare recommends discontinuing the combined contraceptive pill until at least 3 weeks after major surgery.[14]

KEY POINTS
- The combined contraceptive pill carries a small but a real risk of VTE.
- Smoking, hypertension and diabetes increase the risk of VTE with the combined contraceptive pill.
- Combined oral contraceptive (COC) should be prescribed with caution to obese women with a BMI > 30.
- If a thrombophilia screen is positive, the combined contraceptive pill should not be prescribed (absolute contraindication).

References

1 Office for National Statistics. *Opinions Survey Report No. 41: contraception and sexual health, 2008/09* Statistics. Available at: www.statistics.gov.uk/downloads/theme_health/contra2008-9pdf (accessed 10 March 2011).

2 Department of Health. *Venous Thromboembolism (Blood Clot in the Veins) and Third Generation Oral Contraceptive: advice and information from the Department of Health.* Press Release. 2001. Department of health: www.dh.gov.uk:DH (2001).

3 Dinger JC, Heinemann LAJ, Kühl-Habich D. The safety of a drospirenone-containing oral contraceptive: final results from the European Active Surveillance Study on oral contraceptives based on 142,475 women-years of observation. *Contraception.* 2007; **75**(5): 344–54.

4 Guillebaud J. *Contraception Today: a pocketbook for general practitioners.* 5th ed. London: Martin Dunitz; 2004, pp. 20–8.

5 Faculty of Family Planning and Reproductive Health Care, Clinical Effectiveness Unit. *First Prescription of Combined Oral Contraception: recommendations for clinical practice.* July 2006. Available at: www.ffprhc.org.uk/admin/… FirstPrescComboral.ContJan06.pdf (accessed 10 March 2011).

6 Ageno W, Becattini C, Brighton T *et al.* Cardiovascular risk factors and venous thromboembolism: a meta-analysis. *Circulation.* 2008; **117**(1): 93–102.

7 Vandenbroucke JP, Koster T, Briet E *et al.* Increased risk of venous thrombosis in oral-contraceptive users who are carriers of factor V Leiden mutation. *Lancet.* 1994; **344**(8935): 1453–7.

8 Farmer RD, Lawrenson RA, Todd JC *et al.* A comparison of the risks of venous thromboembolic disease in association with different combined oral contraceptives. *Br J Clin Pharmacol.* 2000; **49**(6): 580–90.

9 van Hylckama Vlieg A, Helmerhorst FM, Vandenbrouchke JP *et al.* The venous thrombotic risks of oral contraceptives, effects of oestrogen dose and progestogen type: results of the MEGA case-control study. *BMJ.* 2009; 339: b2921.

10 Lidegaard Ø, Løkkegaard E, Svendsen AL *et al.* Hormonal contraception and risk of venous thromboembolism: national follow-up study. *BMJ.* 2009; 339: b2890.

11 Tanis BC, van den Bosch MA, Kemmeren JM *et al.* Oral contraceptives and the risk of myocardial infarction. *N Engl J Med.* 2001; **345**(25): 1787–93.

12 Kubba A, Guilleband J, Anderson RA *et al.* Contraception. *Lancet.* 2000; **356**(9245): 1913–19.

13 National Institute for Health and Clinical Excellence. *Venous thromboembolism: reducing the risk.* Guideline updates NICE clinical guideline 46 and replaces it. London: NICE; 2010. www.nice.org.uk/nicemedia/pdf/CG92FullGuideline.pdf (accessed 10 March 2011).

14 Faculty of Sexual and Reproductive Healthcare, Clinical Effectiveness Unit. *UK Medical Eligibility Criteria for Contraceptive Use.* London: FSRH; 2009. Available at: www.ffprhc.org.uk/admin/uploads/UKMEC2009.pdf (accessed 10 March 2011).

4

Primary care oral anticoagulant management

Primary care oral anticoagulant management can be as effective as hospital-based clinic. The Birmingham model of primary care anticoagulant management, the only model with a robust evidence, has become an acceptable alternative to hospital outpatient management.[1] This is a nurse-led clinic supervised by a general practitioner using near-patient INR (international normalised ratio) testing and computerised decision support software for support regarding the dose and advice on recall.

In most primary care settings, the blood is taken by a practice/district nurse or healthcare assistant. If a patient is housebound the blood is taken by a community matron/phlebotomist, the sample transported to the hospital clinic for INR estimation[2] and the patient then informed of the result and the dose of warfarin over the telephone.[3]

It is important that, if primary care wishes to provide this service through practice-based commissioning, training, clinical governance and quality assurance procedures are in place.

Most commercially available near-patient INR systems have been evaluated by the regulatory agencies and are found to be accurate. If a device has not had an evaluation it is important that a validation is undertaken locally.

Warfarin

There are various risk assessment tools – a popular one is the CHADS2 score for deciding whether to initiate warfarin.[4]

TABLE 4.1 CHADS2 risk assessment tool

C	Congestive heart failure	1
H	Hypertension or treated hypertension	1
A	Aged 75 years or over	1
D	Diabetes	1
S	Stroke/transient ischaemic attack	1

If the score is 2 or > 2, initiate warfarin.

A major cause of concern in the primary care setting is cognitive impairment of the patient. In this situation it is important to involve the family/carer to make sure that warfarin is taken at the advised dose.

The National Patient Safety Agency (NPSA) anticoagulant alert in 2007 highlighted many risks associated with prescribing of warfarin and how to reduce the risks.[5] The NPSA recommends annual assessment of patients on long-term anticoagulants. One way to avoid errors in general practice is by using proper Read codes:

- 66Q6 – warfarin therapy started
- 66Q – warfarin monitoring
- 66Q5 – warfarin therapy stopped
- 66Q3 – warfarin side effects.

Entering an alert message with the date of initiation and the date of stopping warfarin is another way of alerting other professionals in the primary healthcare team and helping them to reduce the risks.

A recent history of major bleed, malignant hypertension and pregnancy are absolute contraindications. Age alone is no bar as older patients gain most benefit.

Common causes of raised INR[6]

- Concurrent illness (especially if treated with antibiotics).
- Exacerbation of heart failure.

- Incorrect dose of warfarin.
- Concomitant use of a drug that may potentiate the effect of warfarin.
- Binge drinking.

St John's wort and coenzyme Q can affect INR. There have been several case reports of serious interaction resulting in major bleeding with macrolide, best to avoid erythromycin and clindamycin. Broad-spectrum antibiotics eradicate the gut flora and as a result are thought to increase the INR value; however, this effect is only short-lived.

Useful websites with further information on drugs affecting INR include Pharmaceutical Press (www.pharmpress.com) and UK Medicines Information (www.ukmi.nhs.uk).

Alcohol is the most important and common problem. It raises the INR in the short term but lowers it with chronic abuse. It is binge drinking that causes the most acute problems. The patients should be advised either not to drink or to be consistent at all times.

Data from a large registry of patients who were treated with warfarin show that the risk of 30-day bleeding in patients with a single INR measurement between 5.0 and 9.0 is less than 1%.[7]

Management of patients in general practice surgery
Patient with an INR > 4.5 and no sign of bleeding

- Stopping warfarin therapy until the INR comes to a safer level.
- Stopping warfarin and giving low-dose vitamin K.

Evidence from the two randomised controlled trials indicates that, on average, when warfarin therapy is stopped an INR between 6.0 and 10.0 will decline to less than 4.0 in about 2.5 days without vitamin K, and in about 1.4 days with a low-dose oral vitamin K.[8]

When the *INR is between 4.5 and 10.0*, oral vitamin K in a dose of 1.0–2.5 mg will bring the INR level to within therapeutic range in less than 24 hours in two-thirds of the patients.[8]

It seems that low-dose vitamin K may offer an advantage over simply stopping warfarin for a few days. For patients with a history of decompensated heart failure, malignancy or recent surgery and for older patients (especially those who require a weekly dose of warfarin > 15 mg), adding vitamin K may be more appropriate than simple warfarin interruption.[9]

Patients with an INR > 10

These patients should be prescribed a low-dose oral vitamin K of 2.5–5 mg. Quality evidence from cohort studies indicates that this is safe.[10]

Patient receiving warfarin presenting with bleeding

These patients should be referred urgently to the anticoagulant clinic or should be admitted. Bleeding can be life-threatening. Life-threatening bleeding can be a gastrointestinal, intracerebral, genitourinary or retroperitoneal. Bleeding in to an extremity can threaten the functioning of the limb if it causes a compartmental syndrome. Continued bleeding even at a slow rate can further raise the INR as clotting factors are lost with bleeding.

Dabigatran (Pradaxa)

A new oral anticoagulant licensed in 2008 for use in high-risk orthopaedic knee and hip replacement surgery. It is a direct thrombin inhibitor that is taken orally.

Published studies in high-risk elective hip and knee surgery have shown that dabigatran is as effective as low-molecular-weight heparin (LMWH) prophylaxis and can be prescribed for prolonged prophylaxis of up to 14 days after knee surgery and up to 35 days after hip surgery. Dabigatran does not have the risk of heparin-induced thrombocytopenia, which occurs in 0.2–0.5% of patients treated with LMWH.

Dabigatran has shown comparable efficacy with warfarin, in a randomised double-blind trial of patients with acute symptomatic deep-vein thrombosis of the legs or pulmonary embolism. Dabigatran was given in a dose of 150 mg and warfarin was titrated to an international normalised ratio of 2:3 for 6 months, after an initial intravenous anticoagulant, heparin or a low-molecular-weight alternative.[11]

Patients treated with dabigatran do not need their anticoagulation levels monitored and this new drug has additional benefits for the patients as it has no known interactions with food, unlike warfarin.

Prophylaxis should be provided for up to 4 weeks after orthopaedic surgery and can be continued at home after discharge.

In the randomised controlled trial significantly fewer patients had major or clinically relevant non-major bleeds using dabigatran compared with those using warfarin (5.6% versus 8.8%; p-0.002).[11]

It is also much more cost-effective than having a district nurse visit patients at home to administer injectable antithrombotic drugs. Available as 75 mg and 110 mg capsules (cost of both strengths 10 capsules = £21.00 and 60 capsules = £126.00 – price at the time of writing this book).

Rivaroxaban (Xarelto)

Another new oral anticoagulant licensed in 2008 for high-risk orthopaedic knee or hip operations.

Rivaroxaban is a direct factor Xa inhibitor and works at an earlier stage in the coagulation cascade. It does not alter the functions of platelets. Similar to dabigatran, it does not increase the risk of bleeding, unlike LMWH.

It is taken orally once daily, beginning 6–10 hours after surgery. Treatment must continue for 5 weeks after hip surgery (cost of 5 weeks is £157.50 and for 2 weeks after surgery is £63 – at the time of writing this book).

Treatment with rivaroxaban does not require haematological monitoring. Direct comparative trials demonstrated that this drug is at least as effective as the LMWH enoxaparin (Clexane) in preventing thromboembolism.

The above two new oral anticoagulants – dabigatran and rivaroxaban – are in most hospital formularies. The intention is that patients will be discharged into the community after such surgical procedures with prescriptions for extended prophylaxis for up to 35 days. It is hoped that these two drugs will probably become the drug of choice after other moderate- to high-risk major surgery.

KEY POINTS

- In the United Kingdom, two-thirds of all adults admitted to a surgical ward and 40% over the age of 40 years are at risk of venous thromboembolism.[12]
- Primary care can provide a cost-effective oral anticoagulation service with INR monitoring service, preventative steps and follow-up of patients discharged with thrombosis.

- Warfarin is currently the most effective medication for preventing thromboembolic events.
- A recent history of a major bleed and malignant hypertension are absolute contraindications to warfarin.
- Over-the-counter products such as St John's wort and coenzyme Q can affect INR.
- The NPSA recommends annual assessment of patients on long-term warfarin as the risk benefit profile changes regularly.
- Dabigatran is as safe and effective as warfarin for preventing thromboembolism, without the need to monitor blood coagulation.

References

1 Fitzmaurice DA, Hobbs FDR, Murray JA. Monitoring oral anticoagulation in primary care. *BMJ*. 1996; **312**(7044): 1431–2.

2 Baglin T, Luddington R. Reliability of delayed INR determination: implications for decentralized anticoagulant care with off-site blood sampling. *Br J Haematol*. 1997; **96**(3): 431–4.

3 Rodgers H, Sudlow M, Dobson R *et al*. Warfarin anticoagulation in primary care: a regional survey of present practice and clinicians' views. *Br J Gen Pract*. 1997; 47(418): 309–10.

4 Gage BF, Waterman A D, Shannon W *et al*. Validation of clinical classification schemes for predicting stroke: results from the National Registry of Atrial Fibrillation. *JAMA*. 2001; **285**(22): 2864–70.

5 National Patient Safety Agency. *Patient Safety Alert: actions that can make anticoagulant therapy safer*. 28 March 2007. Available at: www.npsa.nhs.uk/EasySiteWeb?GatewayLink.aspx?alld=10797 (accessed 10 March 2011).

6 Panneerselvam S, Baglin C, Lefort W *et al*. Analysis of risk factors for over-anticoagulation in patients receiving long-term warfarin. *Br J Haematol*. 1998; **103**(2): 422–4.

7 Garcia DA, Regan S, Crowther M *et al*. The risk of haemorrhage among patients with warfarin-associated coagulopathy. *J Am Coll Cardiol*. 2006; **47**(4): 804–8.

8 Crowther MA, Julian J, McCarty D *et al*. Treatment of warfarin-associated coagulopathy with oral vitamin K: a randomised controlled trial. *Lancet*. 2000; **356**(9241): 1551–3.

9 Hylek EM, Regan S, Go AS *et al*. Clinical predictors of prolonged delay in

return of the international normalized ratio to within the therapeutic range after excessive anticoagulation with warfarin. *Ann Intern Med.* 2001; **135**(6): 393–400.

10 Gunther KE, Conway G, Leibach L *et al.* Low-dose oral vitamin K is safe and effective for outpatient management of patients with an INR > 10. *Thromb Res.* 2004; **113**(3–4): 205–9.

11 Schulman S, Kearon C, Kakkar AK. Dabigatran versus warfarin in the treatment of acute venous thromboembolism. *N Engl J Med.* 2009; **361**(24): 2342–52.

12 Cohen AT, Tapson VF, Bergmann J-F *et al.* Venous thromboembolism and prophylaxis in the acute hospital care setting (ENDORSE study): a multinational cross-sectional study. *Lancet.* 2008; **371**(9610): 387–94.

5

Prevention of post-operative venous thromboembolism

In 2007 the National Institute for Health and Clinical Excellence (NICE, also NIHCE) published guidance on the prevention of venous thromboembolism (VTE) for surgical patients admitted to hospital.[1] VTE prevention has now been effectively mandated for hospital trusts in the 2010–11 National Health Service Operating Framework and has been declared a national goal for the Commissioning Quality and Innovation (CQUIN) payment framework. The goal is to reduce avoidable deaths and disability. When a trust meets the goal of risk assessment for 90% of all adult inpatients a payment to the trust of 1.5% of the contract value will be triggered.[2,3]

Therefore, a proportion of provider contract value is linked to improvements in venous thromboembolism prevention, in effect mandating this proven best practice.

Recommendations
The following points are recommended for the prevention of post-operative VTE:
- Regard medical patients as being at increased risk of VTE if reduced mobility.
- Regard surgical patients admitted with trauma as at increased risk.

- Regard surgical procedure with a total anaesthetic and surgical time of more than 90 minutes or 60 minutes if the surgery involved the pelvis or lower limb at increased risk.
- Reassess patients within 24 hours of admission and whenever the clinical situation changes.
- Reduce the risks by encouraging patients to become mobile.
- Initiate prophylaxis as soon as possible after risk assessment has been completed and continuing until the patient is no longer at risk.
- Start prophylaxis in patients undergoing elective orthopaedic surgery or surgery for hip fractures, in addition to mechanical stockings with a low-molecular-weight heparin such as enoxaparin (Clexane) or the indirect Factor Xa inhibitor fondaparinux (Arixtra) for 4 weeks, as per NICE guidance.[4]

Following discharge

A large number of procedures are now done as day cases. A study by S Sweetland and colleagues provides a wake-up call for all surgeons and general practitioners. The study investigated a group of middle-aged women at relatively low risk of VTE, without a history of VTE or cancer and who had a single operation as an inpatient or day case. The types of surgery included minor operations and biopsies and more than 60% was day surgery. All types of surgery were associated with increased risk of VTE. The risk was greatest in the first 6 weeks after surgery, peaking in the third week. Risk stayed high for 12 months and was at its maximum between 7 and 12 weeks.[5] This is really important, as most patients receive prophylaxis only while inpatients and the mean inpatient stay for surgical patients is 6 days.[6]

For primary care

- Take note of discharge slip and offer patients and their carers written/verbal information about prophylaxis – that is, name of drug, why started, side effects, interaction and for how long to take.
- Enter an alert message on the computer about the duration of prophylaxis.
- Read coding properly to avoid errors in prescribing and for audit purposes:
  — 8B61, anticoagulant prophylaxis
  — 8B6X, low-dose heparin prophylaxis

- — 66Q, warfarin monitoring
- — 8I71, warfarin not tolerated
- — 66Q4, warfarin dose changed
- — 66Q9, warfarin dose unchanged
- — 66QB, annual warfarin assessment
- — 66QG, INR.
- Use a dedicated anticoagulant template on the computer with headings of warfarin, heparin and other anticoagulants. Each heading can have a drop-down list of drug dose, date started, date stopped and INR monitoring to choose from. Once the medication is stopped it should be removed from the prescribing screen.
- Advise patients on seeking help if any problem arises regarding prophylaxis – who to contact and their contact details.
- Keep yourself and your team up to date by reading NICE guidelines. This can be part of your personal development plan (PDP).

The fact that all types of surgery are at increased risk of DVT means that general practitioners must improve their knowledge about diagnosis and management of this condition.

KEY POINTS
- Out-of-hospital and extended prophylaxis means the primary care team needs to be familiar with up-to-date guidelines.
- Encourage patients to mobilise as soon as possible after discharge.
- Use Read codes in primary care to reduce errors in prescribing.

References

1 Hill J, Treasure T. Reducing the risk of venous thromboembolism (deep vein thrombosis and pulmonary embolism) in inpatients having surgery: summary of NICE guidance. *BMJ.* 2007; **334**(7602): 1053–5.

2 House of Commons Health Committee (2004–05). *The prevention of Venous Thromboembolism in Hospitalised Patients (HC99).*

3 National Institute for Health and Clinical Excellence. *Cost saving guidance.* 5 Aug 2010. Available at: www.nice.org.uk/usingguidance/benefitsofimple mentation/costsavingguidance.Jsp (accessed 10 March 2011).

4 National Institute for Health and Clinical Excellence. *Venous thromboembolism: NICE guideline 46*. London: NIHCE; 2007. Available at www.nice.org.uk/nicemedia/pdf/CG046NICEguideline.pdf (accessed 10 March 2011).

5 Sweetland S, Green J, Liu B *et al.* Duration and magnitude of the postoperative risk of venous thromboembolism in middle aged women: prospective cohort study. *BMJ.* 2009; **339**: b4583.

6 Cohen AT, Tapson VF, Bergman JF *et al.* Venous thromboembolism risk and prophylaxis in the acute hospital care setting (ENDORSE study): a multinational cross-sectional study. *Lancet.* 2008; **371**(9610): 387–94.

6

The diabetic foot

Diabetes UK reports that there is currently a population of 2.8 million known diabetics in the UK.[1] The UK prevalence of diabetes in men aged 65–74 years increased from 5.8% in 1994 to 15.7% in 2006, while that in women increased from 4.8% to 10.4%. Type 2 diabetes is a complex, multi-factorial and progressive metabolic-cardiovascular syndrome. Achieving well-defined targets in type 2 diabetes in the primary care setting is a considerable challenge.

It is estimated that diabetes may be responsible for 5% of total healthcare and 9% of the hospital budgets in the United Kingdom.[2] Diabetics are five times more likely to develop cardiovascular disease, stroke, amputation, blindness and renal failure.[1] Most complications in diabetics are due to poor control and can affect the quality of life,[3] not forgetting the economic and cost implications on the already cash-struggling National Health Service. The foot problem in diabetics can occur in both type 1 and type 2 diabetics. The most at risk are older people and men.[4]

Prevalence

Diabetic foot ulcer prevalence is 4%–10%, with a lifetime risk of 25%.[5] The diabetic foot disease resulting in an amputation has a mortality of 13%–40% at 1 year, rising significantly to 39%–80% at 5 years.[5]

NICE guidelines

In May 2008, the National Institute for Health and Clinical Excellence (NICE, or NIHCE) published new guidelines that highlighted the need to minimise complications combining with a programme promoting healthy lifestyle, stopping smoking and regular exercise.[6] However, for many patients these lifestyle modifications will not be enough to control blood sugar level. Because of the progressive nature of the disease, NICE acknowledges that most patients with type 2 diabetes will eventually require oral anti-diabetes agents to help achieve HbA1c targets, before eventually needing insulin therapy.[6]

It is generally acknowledged that good blood sugar control, combined with cardiovascular risk reduction, can slow the progression of the disease and prevent the development of microvascular complications.[7]

The updated NICE guidelines suggest aiming for an HbA1c target of 6.5% or 7.5% for those at risk of hypoglycaemia.[8] The National Service Framework for diabetes defines poor glycaemic control as HbA1c above 7.5%.[9]

The United Kingdom Prospective Diabetes Study (UKPDS) demonstrated that each 1% reduction in the level of HbA1c reduces the risk of microvascular complications by 37% and diabetes-related death by 21%.[7]

It is recognised that general practitioners (GPs) are well placed to detect and prevent diabetic complications.

Quality and outcomes framework: diabetes indicators

TABLE 6.1 Diabetes mellitus

INDICATOR	POINTS	PAYMENT STAGES
RECORDS		
DM 19 The practice can produce a register of all patients aged 17 years and over with diabetes mellitus, which specifies whether the patient has type 1 or type 2 diabetes.	6	–

(continued)

INDICATOR	POINTS	PAYMENT STAGES

RECORDS

Ongoing management

DM 2	3	40%–90%

The percentage of patients with diabetes whose notes record body mass index in the previous 15 months.

DM 5	3	40%–90%

The percentage of patients with diabetes who have a record of HbA1c or equivalent in the previous 15 months.

DM 23	17	40%–50%

The percentage of patients with diabetes in whom the last HbA1c is 7 or less (or equivalent test/reference range depending on local laboratory) in the previous 15 months.

DM 24	8	40%–70%

The percentage of patients with diabetes in whom the last Hb1Ac is 8 or less (or equivalent test/reference range depending on local laboratory) in the previous 15 months.

DM 25	10	40%–90%

The percentage of patients with diabetes in whom the last HbA1c is 9 or less (or equivalent test/reference range depending on local laboratory) in the previous 15 months.

DM 21	5	40%–90%

The percentage of patients with diabetes who have a record of retinal screening in the previous 15 months.

DM 9	3	40%–90%

The percentage of patients with diabetes with a record of the presence or absence of peripheral pulses in the previous 15 months.

DM 10	3	40%–90%

The percentage of patients with diabetes with a record of neuropathy testing in the previous 15 months.

(*continued*)

INDICATOR	POINTS	PAYMENT STAGES
RECORDS		
DM 11	3	40%–90%
The percentage of patients with diabetes who have a record of blood pressure in the previous 15 months.		
DM 12	18	40%–60%
The percentage of patients with diabetes in whom the last blood pressure is 145/85 mmHg or less.		
DM 13	3	40%–90%
The percentage of patients with diabetes who have a record of microalbuminuria testing in the previous 15 months (exception reporting for patients with proteinuria).		
DM 22	3	40%–90%
The percentage of patients with diabetes who have a record of estimated glomerular filtration rate (eGFR) or serum creatinine testing in the previous 15 months.		
DM 15	3	40%–80%
The percentage of patients with diabetes with a diagnosis of proteinuria or microalbuminuria who are treated with ACE inhibitors (or angiotensin II receptor blockers).		
DM 16	3	40%–90%
The percentage of patients with diabetes who have a record of total cholesterol in the previous 15 months.		
DM 17	6	40%–70%
The percentage of patients with diabetes whose last measured total cholesterol within the previous 15 months is 5 mmol/L or less.		
DM 18	3	40%–85%
The percentage of patients with diabetes who have had influenza immunization in the preceding 1 September to 31 March.		

Source: Quality and Outcomes Framework Guidance for GMS Contract. 2009/10

This document is available in pdf format at www.nhsemployers.org.

Diabetes and the management of the associated cardiovascular risk remain a significant part of the new General Medical Services contract, with 93 points available if all targets are met. Practices achieving HbA1c below 7.5% in 50% of patients with diabetes receive 17 points, and an additional 11 points for achieving HbA1c below 10% in 90% of patients. There are 3 points awarded for neuropathy testing and another 3 points for checking of peripheral pulses.

To achieve these targets in a general practice it is clear that professionals and patients must adopt an intensive approach to management.

The diabetic template on general practice computer systems enables a GP to provide a holistic patient-centred approach to the management of diabetes.

The diabetic template includes:

- recording height, weight, body mass index and waist circumference measurement and advising patients on healthy eating
- recording smoking and alcohol intake and at every attendance encouraging patients to stop
- encouraging self-management and regular self-monitoring of blood sugar
- offering education and reinforcing the advice to attend 6-monthly (if the control is unsatisfactory) or annually (if satisfactory control) for review
- assessing and managing cardiovascular risks such as blood pressure, full lipid profile including low-density lipoprotein (LDL), high-density lipoprotein (HDL) and triglyceride level
- helping achieve and maintain target HbA1c, involving patients in their diabetic control
- ensuring check of kidney function tests, urea and electrolyte check including microalbuminuria
- referring for an annual eye screening either to the primary care trust–led retinal screening service or to a trained and approved optician
- checking feet, use of monofilament, vibration testing and checking pulses for abnormal circulation.

Risk factors

Diabetics with the following risk factors – these factors can lead on to foot complications – must be identified and invited every 6 months for foot check-ups:

- smoker
- older person
- poor mobility
- poor glycaemic control
- past history of foot ulceration
- poor vision, who are unable to care for their own feet
- peripheral vascular disease
- neuropathy.

Pathogenesis

The two main features are neuropathy and ischaemia, both of which pre-dispose to infection. Almost 50% of diabetics over the age of 60 years suffer from diabetic neuropathy, increasing the risk of foot ulceration sevenfold.[10] The neuropathy can be sensory, motor or autonomic. Sensory neuropathy results in failure to perceive damage caused by trauma, which goes unnoticed by the patient until ulceration has ensued. Ulceration of the foot leads to superimposed bacterial infection with Staphylococcus aureus, Streptococcus pyogenes and bacteroides species. Holidays can be a dangerous time for those with neuropathy because of increased risk of injury from walking barefoot on hot beaches or wearing ill-fitting footwear (shoes or sandals). Autonomic neuropathy causes dry skin due to loss of sweating. Muscle atrophy and claw foot deformity are caused by motor neuropathy.

Patients with peripheral vascular disease are predisposed to poor wound healing. Poor glycaemic control in diabetics can also cause poor wound healing. The poorly controlled diabetics are likely to suffer from fungal infections that can lead to skin disruption.[11,12]

Neuropathic pain

Neuropathic pain occurs in 6%–8% of the general population.[13] It is defined as 'pain arising as a direct consequence of a lesion or disease affecting the somato sensory system'.[14] It is common in low socio-economic groups, females and the older population. Apart from diabetes the other causes of neuropathic pains are:

Baron's classification[15]

- Peripheral nervous system (focal and multifocal):
  — post-herpetic neuralgia
  — trigeminal neuralgia
  — post-operative nerve pain, e.g. post-hernia repair
  — post-amputation pain
  — carpal tunnel syndrome.
- Generalised peripheral neuropathies:
  — metabolic, e.g. hypothyroid
  — toxic, e.g. alcohol, chemotherapy
  — vitamin B deficiency
  — infective, e.g. HIV, Guillain–Barré syndrome
  — malignant, e.g. carcinomatous neuropathy.
- Central nervous system lesions:
  — multiple sclerosis
  — spinal cord tumours
  — spinal cord injury
  — brain or spinal cord infarction
  — disc prolapse.

Neuropathic pain has a greater deleterious effect on quality of life than the nociceptive pain.

History

Enquire the history of pain: severity, distribution of pain, aggravating and relieving factors. The classical history of a neuropathic pain is pain arising from an area of altered sensation that may be numb or hyperexcitable.

Hyperalgesia is a response of exaggerated severity following a stimulus such as pinprick.

Allodynia means pain evoked by a stimulus that usually does not cause pain. There are three types of allodynia: thermal (cold/warm), movements and mechanical (static/dynamic).

Hyperpathia is an increased reaction to a painful and often repetitive stimulus.

Ask about sweating, skin temperature, hair or nail changes and muscle weakness or wasting.

Foot examination

Two major complications of diabetes causing foot ulceration are:

- diabetic neuropathy
- abnormal circulation (microvascular and macrovascular).

TABLE 6.2 Diabetes-monitoring Read codes: foot screening

DESCRIPTION	READ CODE
Feet examined	66AE
Diabetic foot examination declined	8I3W
O/E Rt leg pulses present	24E1
O/E absent Rt foot pulses	24EA
O/E Lt leg pulses present	24F1
O/E absent Lt foot pulses	24FA
O/E Rt diabetic foot at risk	2G5A
O/E Rt diabetic foot at low risk	2G5E
O/E Rt diabetic foot at moderate risk	2G5F
O/E Rt diabetic foot at high risk	2G5G
O/E Lt diabetic foot at risk	2G5B
O/E Lt diabetic foot at low risk	2G5I
O/E Lt diabetic foot at moderate risk	2G5J
O/E Lt diabetic foot at high risk	2G5K
O/E Rt diabetic foot ulcerated	2G5H
O/E Lt diabetic foot ulcerated	2G5L
O/E amputated Rt leg	2G42
O/E amputated Lt leg	2G43
Monofilament foot sensation test	311A
10g monofilament sensation present	29B7
10g monofilament sensation absent	29B8
10g monofilament Rt foot normal	29BB
10g monofilament Rt foot abnormal	29B9
10g monofilament Lt foot normal	29BC
10g monofilament Lt foot abnormal	29BA

(continued)

DESCRIPTION	READ CODE
O/E vibration sensation Rt foot normal	29H5
O/E vibration sensation Rt foot abnormal	29H4
O/E vibration sensation Lt foot normal	29H7
O/E vibration sensation Lt foot abnormal	29H6

Equipment

Examination couch, cotton wool to test light sensation, 10 g nylon Semmes–Weinstein monofilament, patella hammer to test knee and ankle jerk, a 128 Hz tuning fork to test vibration perception and a good light source.

Examination

TABLE 6.3 Diabetic foot risk assessment

RISK	CLINICAL EXAMINATION	FOLLOW-UP
Low	Normal pulses Normal sensation	12 months
Increased	Either absent pulses or absent sensation	3–6 months
High	Either absent pulses or neuropathy plus skin changes Previous ulceration	3 months
Ulcerated foot	Ulcer	Refer immediately

- The patient should be examined lying down on an examination couch with a good light source.
- Shoes, socks (tights or stockings) must be removed.
- *Inspection*: the upper and lower surfaces of feet, nails and heels must be inspected carefully. Look for colour, dryness, corns, callosities, deformities, any evidence of infection (fungal/bacterial), cellulitis and any ingrowing toe nail (IGTN). Nail-cutting technique should be looked at and noted.
- *Palpation*: dorsalis pedis and posterior tibial should be palpated in all diabetics. If severe ischaemia is suspected, all lower-limb pulses should be palpated.

- *Pressure sensation check*: this is done by placing the 10 g monofilament at a right angle to the skin on the planter surface of the foot. The pressure is applied until the filament buckles (indicating that enough pressure has been applied). Inability to perceive the 10 g force is associated with clinically significant large fibre neuropathy.[16] Validated tools must be used to assess neuropathic pain – for example, the Leeds Assessment of Neuropathic Symptoms and Signs (LANNS).[17] Or the painDETECT questionnaire.[18] These tools have about 80% accuracy but cannot replace good clinical examination. Clinical assessment must include examining and comparing the affected area with an unaffected contralateral side. Light stroking may show allodynia. Inability to differentiate cold and warm suggests alteration in thermal thresholds.
- *Vibration sense check*: this is tested with a 128 Hz tuning fork placed on the bony prominence of the big toe.
- *Biothesiometer*: this is an electrical device that assesses vibration perception threshold. A threshold of more than 25V has a sensitivity of 83% for predicting foot ulcer over a period of 4 years.[19]
- *ABPI measurement*: this is discussed in Chapter 10.

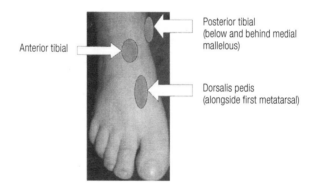

Anterior tibial

Posterior tibial
(below and behind medial mallelous)

Dorsalis pedis
(alongside first metatarsal)

FIGURE 6.1 Checking foot pulsation

Neuropathic ulcer
- Painless ulcer.
- Located on the sole of the foot under the metatarsal heads and the ball of the foot.
- Foot is warm to touch.
- Punched-out ulcer.

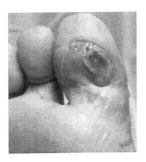

FIGURE 6.2 Neuropathic ulcer

- A rim of callus around the ulcer.
  Refer a neuropathic ulcer to the specialist.

Examination of shoes
Shoes should be examined inside and outside for:
- depth
- width
- heel
- insoles.

Examination of socks/tights
They must be examined and patient advised on:
- correct fit
- material (cotton)
- advice on wearing inside out (seams on the outside)
- no use of garters
- no biological washing powder (it can be irritating to the skin).

Charcot's foot
This is a rare complication of diabetes associated with disorganisation of the bony architecture of the foot. The resulting deformity creates areas of pressure that are predisposed to callus formation. This foot is at an increased risk of ulceration and warrants immediate referral.[20] During the acute stage the foot is painful and swollen and can be misdiagnosed as cellulitis.

Management

Treating painful diabetic neuropathy (PDN) can be challenging in primary care. It is important for the primary care physician to assess the severity of the condition based on symptoms and clinical examination.

Optimising glycaemic control is very important. Large fluctuations in blood sugar level can exacerbate neuropathic pain.[21]

An ulcerated foot should be referred urgently to the diabetic clinic in the secondary care. A patient with absent pulsations and evidence of neuropathy remains at a high risk of ulcer and must be followed up 3-monthly, either in the surgery or at home (if housebound).

A low-risk patient with normal pulses and normal sensation can be seen every 12 months.

PDN care pathway

About a third of patients with chronic neuropathic pain do not receive any treatment.[22]

Treatment must be both non-pharmacological and pharmacological.

Non-pharmacological treatment

- Heat and cold therapy.
- Ultrasound.
- TENS – transcutaneous electrical nerve stimulation.
- Acupuncture.
- Nerve block.
- Psychological therapy – cognitive behavioural therapy.

It is important to assess the patient's expectations against the medical evidence for these strategies.

Pharmacological treatment

This is an important part of treatment in a primary care setting. A patient presenting with symptoms of neuropathic pain expects a form of medication for pain control from his or her GP.

Effective pain relief with a single drug is achieved in less than 50% of patients with neuropathic pain.[23]

It is usual to start with monotherapy, but there may be a need to move on to a combination therapy if pain control is not achieved.

It is safer to start with the low dose, titrating the dose depending on the clinical response but to be guided by the side effects. There must be at least 2 weeks at the maximum tolerated dose before changing to another formulation.

It often requires several consultations with the GP, which sometimes can be done over the telephone. A written instruction sheet with guidance about the dose increase and side effects can cut down on unnecessary surgery consultation.

The patient must be warned that the goal is pain control, not pain cure.

GPs should treat PDN according to the algorithm based on NICE guidance.[24]

First-line treatment

Always start at a lower dose, titrating it upwards to an effective dose or the patient's maximum tolerated dose.

- Oral duloxetine starting with 60 mg/day, maximising to 120 mg/day.
- If oral duloxetine contraindicated, try amitriptyline starting with 10 mg/day, maximising to 75 mg/day.
- If patient is experiencing side effects with amitriptyline, try nortriptyline or imipramine.

First-line treatment (unsatisfactory pain control with maximum tolerated dose with first-line treatment)

- Switch over to amitriptyline (nortriptyline or imipramine if side effects with amitriptyline) *or* pregabalin starting with 150 mg/day (divided into two doses) maximising to 600 mg/day (divided into two doses), if first-line treatment was duloxetine.
- Switch to duloxetine *or* pregabalin if amitriptyline was the first-line.

Second-line treatment (unsatisfactory pain control with maximum tolerated dose with second-line treatment)

- Strong opioids are effective in neuropathic pain and may be required. They should be used according to the British Pain Society guidelines on prescribing.[25]
- Referral to pain clinic.
- While waiting for referral try tramadol in a dose of 50–100 mg every

4 hours, titrating slowly depending upon the pain relief to a maximum dose of 400 mg/day *or* the combination of tramadol with amitriptyline *or* duloxetine.

- Topical lidocaine for people unable to take oral medication.
- Lidocaine 5% patches can be used for localised areas of pain, especially if there is allodynia.

Pain clinic referral

Consider referral to pain clinic specialist at any stage, including at initial presentation and at the time of clinical review if there is:

- severe pain
- pain causing limitation of daily activities
- deterioration of underlying health condition.

Infected ulcer

- Always take a swab for culture and sensitivity.
- Use cefalexin, clindamycin or co-amoxiclav while waiting for the wound swab results.
- If no response *or* severe infection, patient should be admitted for intravenous antibiotics.

KEY POINTS

- Good glycaemic control remains the cornerstone of treatment to reduce the complication of PDN.
- GPs have a key role in identifying those at risk of developing foot complications.
- PDN should be treated according to the algorithm based on NICE guidance.
- Start with monotherapy, but move on to combination therapy quickly if pain control is not achieved.
- Consideration should be given to patient empowerment to encourage adherence to drug regimes.

References

1 Diabetes UK. www.diabetes.org.uk (accessed 10 March 2011).

2 Department of Health (DoH). *Turning the Corner: improving diabetes care.* DoH; 13 June 2006.

3 Jermendy G, Hungarian RECAP Group, Erdesz D *et al.* Outcomes of adding second hypoglycemic drug after metformin monotherapy failure among type 2 diabetes in Hungary. *Health Qual Life Outcomes.* 2008; **6**: 88.

4 Rathur HM, Boulton AJ. The diabetic foot. *Clin Dermatol.* 2007; **25**(1): 109–20.

5 Singh N, Armstrong DG, Lipsky BA. Preventing foot ulcers in patients with diabetes. *JAMA.* 2005; **293**(2): 217–28.

6 National Institute for Health and Clinical Excellence. *Type 2 diabetes – the management of type 2 diabetes: NICE guideline 66.* London: NIHCE; 2008. www.bmj.com/content/336/7656/1306.full.pdf (accessed 10 March 2011).

7 Stratton IM, Adler AI, Neil HA *et al.* Association of glycaemia with macrovascular and microvascular complications of type 2 diabetes (UKPDS 35): prospective observational study. *BMJ.* 2000; **321**(7258): 405–12.

8 National Institute for Health and Clinical Excellence. *Type 2 diabetes: the management of type 2 diabetes. Newer agents for blood glucose control in type 2 diabetes; NICE guideline 87.* London: NIHCE; 2009. http://guidance.nice.org.uk/CG87 (accessed 10 March 2011).

9 Department of Health (DoH). *National Service Framework for Diabetes Standards.* London: The Stationery Office; 2001.

10 Young MJ, Boulton AJ, MacLeod AF *et al.* A multicentre study of the prevalence of diabetic peripheral neuropathy in the United Kingdom hospital clinic population. *Diabetologia.* 1993; **36**(2): 150–4.

11 Geerlings SE, Hoepelman AI. Immune dysfunction in patients with diabetes mellitus (DM). *FEMS Immunol Med Microbiol.* 1999; **26**(3–4): 259–65.

12 Gupta AK, Humke S. The prevalence and management of onychomycosis in diabetic patients. *Eur J Dermatol.* 2000; **10**(5): 379–84.

13 Torrance N, Smith BH, Bennett MI *et al.* The epidemiology of chronic pain of predominantly neuropathic origin: results from a general population survey. *J Pain.* 2006; **7**(4): 281–9.

14 Treede RD, Jensen TS, Campbell JN *et al.* Neuropathic pain: redefinition and a grading system for clinical and research purposes. *Neurology.* 2008; **70**(18): 1630–5.

15 Baron R. Mechanisms of disease: neuropathic pain; a clinical perspective. *Nat Clin Pract Neurol.* 2006; **2**(2): 95–106.

16 Armstrong DG. The 10-g monofilament: the diagnostic divining rod for the diabetic foot? *Diabetes Care.* 2000; **23**(7): 887.

17 Bennett M. The LANSS Pain Scale: the Leeds assessment of neuropathic symptoms and signs. *Pain.* 2001: **92**(1–2): 147–57.

18 Freynhagen R, Baron R, Gockel U *et al.* painDETECT: a new screening questionnaire to identify neuropathic components in patients with back pain. *Curr Med Res Opin.* 2006; **22**(10): 1911–20.

19 Young MJ, Breddy JL, Veves A *et al.* The prediction of diabetic neuropathic foot ulceration using vibration perception thresholds: a prospective study. *Diabetes Care.* 1994; **17**(6): 557–60.

20 Jude EB, Boulton AJ. Update on Charcot neuroarthropathy. *Curr Diab Rep.* 2001; **1**(3): 228–32.

21 Wong MC, Chung JW, Wong TK. Effects of treatment for symptoms of painful diabetic neuropathy: systematic review. *BMJ.* 2007; **335**(7610): 87.

22 Finnerup NB, Otto M, McQuay HJ *et al.* Algorithm for neuropathic pain treatment: an evidence based proposal. *Pain* 2005; **118**(3): 289–305.

23 Eisenberg E, McNicol ED, Carr DB. Efficacy and safety of opioid agonists in the treatment of neuropathic pain of nonmalignant origin: systematic review and meta-analysis of randomized controlled trials. *JAMA.* 2005; **293**(24): 3043–52.

24 National Institute for Health and Clinical Excellence. *Neuropathic Pain: the pharmacological management of neuropathic pain in adults in non-specialist settings; NICE guideline 96.* London: NIHCE; 2010. www.nice.org.uk/guidance/CG96 (accessed 10 March 2011).

25 British Pain Society. *Opioids for persistent pain: Good practice.* (2005) 388–95. Available at: www.britishpainsociety.org/book_opioid_main.pdf (accessed 10 March 2011).

Restless legs syndrome

Restless legs syndrome (RLS) was first described by an English Physician, Sir Thomas Willis, in London in 1672.[1] The term 'restless legs' was introduced by the Swedish Neurologist Karl A Ekbom in 1945.[2] Ekbom was not clear about the cause of the condition although in some publications he emphasised iron deficiency anaemia as a major contributory factor. In his paper, Ekbom described two types of RLS:

1 *asthenia crurum paraesthetica* (sensory form).
2 *asthenia crurum dolorosa* (painful form).[1]

Definition

The International Restless Legs Syndrome Study Group (IRLSSG)[3] defines minimum diagnostic criteria for RLS as:

- desire to move limbs, usually associated with paraesthesia/dysaesthesia
- motor restlessness during sleep
- the presence of symptoms that either worsen or exist exclusively at rest – partial/temporary relief with activity
- symptoms worse in the evening or at night.

Additional but not obligatory criteria:

- sleep disturbance with tiredness during the day
- periodic limb movements
- positive family history
- a normal neurological examination

- chronic symptoms with remissions and exacerbations
- dopamine responsiveness.

Epidemiology

RLS is under-diagnosed and under-treated.[4] Recent studies, utilising the IRLSSG criteria, showed a general prevalence of RLS between 5% and 15%. The condition increases with age. In an international study the prevalence of RLS was 8.7% in the 70–79 age group, 4.7% in the 40–49 age group and 2.7% in the 15–19 age group.[5]

There are about 5 million people affected by RLS in the United Kingdom.[6]

A study in Singapore found a rather low prevalence in the Asian population: only 0.1% in those aged over 21 years and 0.6% in those aged over 55 years.[7] There is a strong genetic linkage to RLS. The genetic linkage has been reported on 9, 12 and 14 chromosomes.[8,9] It may affect children and adolescents,[10] and patients with early onset of the condition often have a strong family history of it.[11]

Aetiology

RLS may present in either a primary or secondary form. Primary (idiopathic RLS) has an associated family history in over 60% of cases, often with an autosomal dominant inheritance.[12]

The most common cause of secondary RLS is iron deficiency anaemia. Evidence suggests a link with iron metabolism and the dopamine/opiate neurotransmitter pathways.[13]

Iron metabolism has a circadian rhythm, similar to dopamine, and is interlinked with dopamine pathways in the brain. There is a possible association between RLS and hypothyroidism, rheumatoid arthritis and diabetes. It is also frequently associated with uraemia, seen in up to 50% of renal dialysis patients.[14] Certain drugs may also cause RLS; these include lithium, tricyclic antidepressants and metoclopramide.

Diagnosis

The diagnosis is essentially clinical. A good and thorough history from the patient/partner/carer is all that is required.

Discomfort in the legs is a typical early feature. The crucial feature of this syndrome is the unpleasant and irresistible urge to move the legs while sitting or lying down.

The patient may find it difficult to describe the symptoms. The most commonly used words include *creeping, crawling, burning, tingling, aching* or *cramp-like sensations.* The symptoms are uncomfortable and unpleasant. Generally the symptoms are in both legs and mainly in the thighs and calves rather than the feet.

The upper limbs can be affected in up to half of the patients.[15]

The symptoms are worse in the evening and at night, with a peak onset between midnight and 4 a.m. There is a mild relief of the symptoms on moving the legs.

It is common for a patient to get out of bed and walk around. Interrupted sleep causes physical, mental and emotional tiredness.

Periodic leg movements (PLMs) are common in RLS and are repetitive. There is associated fanning of the small toes, extension of the big toe and flexion at the ankles and knees. PLMs usually occur during sleep, causing sleep disturbance. In one study 95% of patients with RLS reported sleep problems.[16]

The speed of onset of the symptoms varies, with the majority describing it as a gradual progression but others describing more of an acute onset. The majority of cases of acute and subacute onset belong to secondary RLS due to iron deficiency anaemia or uraemia.

Clinical examination

This is completely normal unless there are features of secondary causes of RLS. It is important to do a vascular and neurological examination to exclude vascular and neurological problems.

Laboratory investigations

Unfortunately, there are no laboratory tests to diagnose RLS. It is, however, necessary to obtain a full blood count, ferritin level and B_{12} and folate levels. Diabetes mellitus and uraemia should be excluded by doing a fasting blood sugar, urea and electrolytes. Patients with severe symptoms and sleep problems may require sleep studies such as polysomnography.

Differential diagnosis

a. *Trapped nerve, poor circulation or arthritis.* In primary care RLS is mis-diagnosed as trapped nerve, poor circulation or arthritis. Patients with peripheral arterial disease will describe intermittent claudication on walking that is relieved by rest. *Neurogenic claudication* due to stenosis of the lumbar canal is relieved by sitting.

   Not one of these conditions would satisfy the IRLSSG criteria for diagnosis of RLS.[17]

b. *Meralgia paraesthetica.* This is a condition confused with RLS. This is also common in old age but associated with pain and paraesthesiae in the distribution of the lateral femoral cutaneous nerve of the thigh.[18]

   Akathisia is a form of motor restlessness related to neuroleptic drug intake and is common in Parkinson's disease, in both the treated and the untreated form. In this condition there is no diurnal variation. The patient is constantly changing position from sitting to standing or walking.[18]

c. *Attention deficit hyperactivity disorder in children.*

d. *Anxiety disorder.*

e. *Intermittent claudication.*

f. *Nocturnal leg cramps.*

Treatment

Non-pharmacological

- Reassurance is a very important part of the management and usually all that is required in mild RLS.
- Lifestyle changes by reducing alcohol and caffeine intake such as tea, coffee, chocolate and soft drinks. Similarly, cutting down or stopping smoking can also be beneficial.
- Aerobic exercises, walking and stretching exercises in moderation can be helpful, although overdoing it can sometimes exacerbate the symptoms. Similarly, relaxation exercises, yoga, massaging the affected limbs and aromatherapy may be beneficial, though there is a lack of evidence that this works.[18] Applying hot or cold packs can be helpful.
- Dietary or prescription medication of iron if low ferritin level.
- Good sleep hygiene – having a hot bath before sleep, having a warm milky drink and enjoying relaxation/soothing music.

- Ask the patient to join a support group. The Ekbom Support Group website provides information for patients on restless legs syndrome (www.ekbom.org.uk/).

Top tips during an attack:
- walking or undertaking an activity as a distraction[18]
- massaging the limb
- keeping the mind actively engaged, either by reading a novel or listening to music.

Pharmacological

Drug treatment should be reserved for more severe cases. Patients with disturbed sleep causing daytime tiredness and inability to cope with day-time tasks should be treated. A general guide for which patients with RLS symptoms to treat is:[3]
- symptoms lasting for more than two weeks
- disturbed sleep (< 5 hours of sleep)
- relationship/marital stress
- waking more than three times per night because of RLS symptoms
- affecting next-day activities.

Severe symptoms that require drug treatment occur in 20%–25% of patients with RLS.[19]

Medication should be started in a low dose and titrated upwards gradually, depending upon the response.[20–22] The patient should be advised to take the medication 1–2 hours before sleep time. The following factors should be taken into consideration when deciding which drug to use:
- severity of symptoms – in some cases the patient may require a combination of drugs from different groups
- age of the patient
- pregnancy – RLS in pregnancy should not be treated and patients can be reassured that it is likely to resolve completely after the delivery
- renal failure.

Some drugs can cause worsening of RLS and should be avoided:
- diuretics
- beta blockers

- lithium
- calcium antagonists
- phenytoin
- some antihistamines
- tranquillisers.

Drug withdrawal may be an option in these patients.
Dopaminergic drugs are the single and useful form of therapy.[23]

- Start treatment with a dopamine non-ergot agonist such as pramipexole (Mirapexin) or ropinirole (Adartrel) given at night. Dopamine agonists have a longer half-life than levodopa with reduced risk of rebound.[24]
- Both pramipexole and ropinirole are equally effective and licensed in the United Kingdom for RLS. The dose for pramipexole is 0.125 mg in the evening, increasing at weekly intervals to 0.25 mg, 0.5 mg or 0.75 mg if needed. The recommended dose for ropinirole is 0.25 mg to be given at night, increasing only if required at weekly intervals to 0.5 mg, 1.0 mg, 1.5 mg or 2.0 mg as a single dose. The majority of patients respond to a low dose of either drug.
- Levodopa, 100–600 mg taken at bedtime, may be used if patients are intolerant to dopamine agonists. Several studies have demonstrated the effectiveness of levodopa.[25] However, it has a relatively short half-life and does not provide sufficient night cover. Up to 80% of patients treated with levodopa experience augmentation or rebound; therefore, long-term use is limited. Levodopa is useful for intermittent RLS. Anorexia, nausea and vomiting are the most common side effects. Levodopa and dopamine agonists should be used with caution in patients with angle-closure glaucoma, cardiac or peptic ulcer disease.
- Alternative dopamine agonists such as bromocriptine, pergolide or cabergoline can be tried if pramipexole or ropinirole are not effective. If patients have rebound phenomenon (early morning symptoms) or augmentation (evening/daytime spreading to upper limbs), dopamine agonists can be given in three divided doses.
- An antiepileptic such as carbamazepine (single or divided doses, 100–600 mg) or gabapentin (300–2400 mg, in three divided doses) can be tried in resistant cases. These drugs work by inhibiting hyperactivity

in the nervous system that may be related to the symptoms. Gabapentin is particularly useful in patients with painful RLS.

- Patients with severe sleep problems should be treated with zopiclone in a dose of 3.75 mg increasing to 7.5 mg or clonazepam 0.5–2 mg in the evening.
- Oxycodone can be used in the dose of 2.5mg to 25 mg in painful RLS.
- Tramadol in the dose of 50–100 mg can be tried in patients with painful RLS and insomnia.

TABLE 7.1 Restless legs syndrome[20–22,26]

AGENT	ADVANTAGES	DISADVANTAGES
Dopaminergic agent Levodopa	Can be used on a p.r.n. basis	GI upset Hallucination Hypotension Arrhythmia
Dopamine agonists Prampipexole Ropinirole	Moderate to severe restless legs syndrome	Nausea Orthostatic hypotension Somnolence
Opiods Codine Tramadol Oxycodone	p.r.n./daily	Constipation Tolerance Dependance
Benzodiazepine Temazepam Clonazepam	To improve sleep	Daytime sleepiness Cognitive impairment in older people
Iron	If ferritin is low	GI upset

Refractory RLS

Patients with refractory symptoms could benefit by:

- adding another medication, e.g. adding a drug from other class to the current dopamine agonist
- trying a different class of dopamine agonist drug
- switching over to an opioid; however, opioids have a problem with addiction and tolerance and should be used for resistant and severe symptomatic patients.

When to refer

- Treatment failure.
- Not sure about the diagnosis.
- Severe refractory patients.

KEY POINTS

- RLS is a common condition but, despite its prevalence, remains under-diagnosed.
- Patients with early onset often have a family history of the condition.
- Most patients do not require any treatment.
- In severe cases dopamine agonists should be prescribed.
- Must exclude iron deficiency anaemia.

References

1 Willis T. *De anima brutorum*. London: Wells Scott; 1672.

2 Ekbom KA. Restless legs syndrome. *Acta Med Scand*. 1945; 158: 4–122.

3 Allen RP, Picchietti D, Hening WA *et al*. Restless legs syndrome: diagnostic criteria, special considerations and epidemiology; a report from the restless legs syndrome diagnostic and epidemiology workshop at the National Institutes of Health. *Sleep Med*. 2003; **4**(2): 101–19.

4 Medcalf P, Bhatia KP. Restless legs syndrome. *BMJ*. 2006; **333**(7566): 457–8.

5 Ohayon MM, Roth T. Prevalence of restless legs syndrome and periodic limb movement disorder in the general population. *J Psychosom Res*. 2002; **53**(1): 547–54.

6 Rothdach AJ, Trenkwalder C, Haberstock J *et al*. Prevalence and risk factors of RLS in an elderly population: the MEMO study. Memory and Morbidity in Augsburg Elderly. *Neurology*. 2005; **54**(5): 1064–8.

7 Tan EK, Seah A, See SJ, *et al*. Restless legs syndrome in an Asian population: a study in Singapore. *Mov Disord*. 2001; **16**(3): 577–9.

8 Chokroverty S, Jankovic J. Restless legs syndrome: a disease in search of identity. *Neurology*. 1999; **52**(5): 907–10.

9 Dhawan V, Ali M, Chaudhuri KR. Genetic aspects of restless legs syndrome. *Postgrad Med J*. 2006; **82**(972): 626–9.

10 Walters AS, Picchietti DL, Ehrenberg BL *et al*. Restless legs syndrome in childhood and adolescence. *Pediatr Neurol*. 1994; **11**(3): 241–5.

11 Godbout R, Montplaisir J, Poirier G. Epidemiological data in familial restless legs syndrome. *Sleep Res.* 1987; 16: 228.

12 Trenkwalder C, Seidel VC, Gasser T *et al.* Clinical symptoms and possible anticipation in a large kindred of familial restless legs syndrome. *Mov Disord.* 1996; **11**(4): 389–94.

13 Allen R. Dopamine and iron in the pathophysiology of restless legs syndrome (RLS). *Sleep Med.* 2004; 5(4): 385–91.

14 Winkleman JW, Chertow GM, Lazarus JM. Restless legs syndrome in end-stage renal disease. *Am J Kidney Dis.* 1996; **28**(3): 372–8.

15 Montplaisir J, Boucher S, Poirier G *et al.* Clinical, polysomnographic, and genetic characteristics of restless legs syndrome: a study of 133 patients diagnosed with new standard criteria. *Mov Disord.* 1997; **12**(1): 61–5.

16 Winkleman J, Wetter TC, Collado-Seidel V *et al.* Clinical characteristics and frequency of the hereditary restless legs syndrome in a population of 300 patients. *Sleep.* 2000; **23**(5): 597–602.

17 Muzerengi S, Lewis H, Chaudhuri KR. Restless legs syndrome: a review of diagnosis and management. *Int J Sleep Disord.* 2006; **1**(2): 34–46.

18 MacMahon D, Muzerengi S, Chaudhuri KR. Treatment and identification of restless legs syndrome. Prescriber. 2008; 19(3)56–59. Available at http://onlinelibrary.wiley.com/doi/10.1002/psb.190/abstract.

19 Chaudhuri KR. The restless legs syndrome: time to recognize a very common movement disorder. *Pract Neurol.* 2003; 3: 204–13.

20 O'Keeffe ST. Restless legs syndrome: a review. *Arch Intern Med.* 1996: **156**(3): 243–8.

21 Hening W, Allen R, Earley C *et al.* The treatment of restless legs syndrome and periodic limb movement disorder: an American Academy of Sleep Medicine Review. *Sleep.* 1999; **22**(7): 970–99.

22 Comella C. Restless legs syndrome: treatment with dopaminergic agents. *Neurology.* 2002; **58**(4 Suppl. 1); S87–92.

23 Schapira AH. Restless legs syndrome: an update on treatment options. *Drugs.* 2004; **64**(2): 149–58.

24 Trenkwalder C, Stiasny-Kolster K, Kupsch A *et al.* Controlled withdrawal of pramipexole after 6 months of open-label treatment in patients with restless legs syndrome. *Mov Disord.* 2006; **21**(9): 1404–10.

25 Akpinar S. Treatment of restless legs syndrome with levodopa plus benserazide. *Arch Neurol.* 1982; **39**(11): 739.

26 National Centre on Sleep Disorders Research. National Heart, Lung and

Blood Institute and National Institute of Health (NIH). *Restless Legs Syndrome: detection and management in primary care.* 2000; NIH publication No 00-3788.

8

Intermittent claudication

Definition

Intermittent claudication (Latin: *claudicatio intermittens*) is defined as pain in the legs that is brought on by exercise and relieved by rest. This is the most commonly presented symptom of peripheral vascular disease.

The word '*claudication*' is derived from the Latin *claudicare* meaning 'to limp' and is associated with the Roman Emperor Claudius, who was said to walk with a limp.

Incidence

It affects between 1.7% and 7.1% of people over the age of 55 years.[1] The incidence increases with age.[2]

Morbidity and mortality

IC is a benign symptom with only 2% of patients requiring a major amputation. It is a powerful marker of increased cardiovascular risk.[3] Twenty to thirty per cent of patients with IC will not survive past 5 years due to cardiovascular events.[4]

Not only the symptomatic patients but also the asymptomatic patients suffer from increased risk due to cardiovascular events.

The first aim and objective should be identifying these patients and treating them appropriately to reduce the cardiovascular risk.[5]

Diagnosis

History

The patient presents with a history of pain in the calves after exercise. The calf muscles are the most common site of claudication but it can also occur in the thigh or buttock muscles if there is more proximal blockage. During exercise there is a build up of lactic acid due to anaerobic respiration if the oxygen demand is not met due to arterial blockage. It is the accumulation of the lactic acid that causes pain. The pain disappears usually within less than 5 minutes, when the patient stops and rests, only to reoccur when the patient starts walking again.

In spinal cord claudication, pain is localised to a muscle group and on walking there is a history of weakness, numbness or heaviness rather than pain.

The Edinburgh Claudication Questionnaire

This is a simple screening tool for diagnosing IC. This is simple enough and can be used in the primary care setting.

TABLE 8.1 The Edinburgh Claudication Questionnaire

EDINBURGH CLAUDICATION QUESTIONNAIRE	POSITIVE CLAUDICANT
1 Do you get pain/discomfort in your leg(s) when you walk?	
▪ Yes	YES
▪ No	
▪ I am unable to walk	
If you answered 'yes' to question 1 please answer the following questions; otherwise, you need not continue.	
2 Does this pain ever begin when you are standing still/ sitting?	
▪ Yes	NO
▪ No	
3 Do you get the pain if you walk uphill or hurry?	
▪ Yes	YES
▪ No	

(continued)

EDINBURGH CLAUDICATION QUESTIONNAIRE	POSITIVE CLAUDICANT
4 Do you get it when you walk at an ordinary pace on the level?	
▪ Yes	YES (grade 1)
▪ No	NO (grade 2)
5 What happens to it if you stand still?	
▪ Usually continues more than 10 minutes	Disappears in
▪ Usually disappears in 10 minutes or less	10 minutes or less
6 Where do you get the pain/discomfort?	
▪ Claudication pain typically occurs in the calf regardless of whether pain is also in other sites. Atypical claudication is pain in the buttock or thigh in the absence of any calf pain. The pain in the shins, joints, feet or hamstrings, in the absence of any calf pain, excludes intermittent claudication.	

Examination

The patient with claudication symptoms should have peripheral pulses checked. Absence of pulses in the ipsilateral leg gives a clue to the diagnosis.

Feet should be examined for ulcers, particularly in patients with diabetes.

Ankle Brachial Pressure Index

The Ankle Brachial Pressure Index (ABPI, *see* Chapter 10) can be measured using a handheld Doppler. An ABPI < 0.9 is indicative of peripheral vascular disease.

Risk factors

- Smoking.
- Hypertension.
- Diabetes.
- Hypercholesterolemia.
- Elevated level of fibrinogen.

69

Severity of peripheral arterial disease

The Fontaine classification is a simple method of classifying the severity of the disease as four stages. These stages are:

1 asymptomatic
2 intermittent claudication
3 rest pain
4 tissue loss.

Stages 3 and 4 are also called *critical ischaemia* as amputation is threatened. All patients should be treated with risk reduction therapy.

www.dwp.gov.uk/publications/...a-z-of.../fontaine-pvd.shtml

Referral to secondary care

The primary care physician can play a major role in diagnosing and managing IC. Even though it is not included in the Quality and Outcomes Framework and there is no target incentive, general practitioners (GPs) are involved in assessing cardiovascular risks in all patients over the age of 40 years and managing these as part of a locally enhanced scheme.

Diabetes is included in the General Medical Services (GMS) contract and has a target payment towards control of blood pressure, cholesterol and circulatory assessment.

There are three main criteria for referral to secondary care:

- diagnosis in doubt
- major impairment of quality of life despite appropriate management
- Fontaine classification stages 3 and 4.

Management

- Smoking cessation.
- Regular exercise.
- Weight reduction.
- Management of hypertension.
- Management of diabetes.
- Antiplatelet therapy.
- Drug therapy.
- Vascular interventions.

See Chapter 11 (The management of Peripheral arterial disease in primary care) and Chapter 12 (Tackling smoking: role of the GP).

Exercise

There is general agreement that exercise is of benefit to people with IC. Regular exercise should be encouraged to increase walking distance and cardiovascular health.[6] The most effective is three supervised walking sessions a week on a treadmill – the patient should be encouraged to walk through pain. Over a period of 1 hour the patient is encouraged to walk to near-maximal pain, then stop till pain is relieved and then start walking again to near-maximal pain.[7]

A referral to a health trainer or exercise on prescription is useful if available in your area. These services are expensive and the primary care trust may not be willing to provide this free of charge. To motivate a patient to join a gym can be difficult in a real-world situation.

Weight reduction

All patients should be given a weight reduction diet sheet. Encourage patients to eat less saturated fat, reduce salt intake and eat five portions of fruit and vegetables a day and more oily fish. Drugs like orlistat (lipase inhibitor) can be prescribed if patient has a body mass index (BMI) of $30 \, kg/m^2$ or more *or* in patients with a BMI of $28 \, kg/m^2$ in the presence of other risk factors. Orlistat should be used in conjunction with other lifestyle measures. Patient must lose half a kg per week to justify another prescription. The treatment can be continued beyond 12 weeks if the patient has lost 5% or more of the initial weight.

Management of hypertension

Blood pressure should be treated to a target of 140/90 as recommended by NICE/BHS.[13] NICE recommends that drug treatment should be offered when blood pressure reaches 160/100mm Hg with the aim of reducing it to below 140/90mm Hg.[14] Beta blockers should not be used in these patients.

An ACE (angiotensin-converting enzyme) inhibitor should be the first choice. If the patient develops a cough an ARBs (angiotensin-II receptor blockers) should be considered.

The Heart Outcomes Prevention Evaluation (HOPE) study showed that

ACE inhibitor ramipril reduces morbidity and mortality in patients with peripheral arterial disease by around 25%.[8]

Antiplatelet therapy

All patients should be given low-dose soluble aspirin (75 mg) unless side effects not tolerated or contraindicated.

In these patients clopidogrel (75 mg) should be prescribed.

The Antithrombotic Trialists' (ATT) Collaboration is an impressive meta-analysis of 16 secondary and 6 primary prevention trials of long-term aspirin therapy versus control. This included 17,000 secondary and 95,000 primary prevention patients. The results showed that in secondary prevention trials, low dose aspirin significantly reduced the absolute risk of major vessel events – 6.7% per year versus 8.2% per year in controls. There was a significant reduction in stroke but with no significant increase in haemorrhagic stroke. In primary prevention without previous disease, aspirin is of uncertain value.[11]

Drug therapy

Drugs used in patients with IC are:
- cilostazol
- pentoxifylline (oxpentifylline)
- naftidrofuryl.

Cilostazol is probably the first-line drug of choice in selected patients, given in a dose of 100 mg twice daily. It is generally well tolerated.[9] The contraindications are severe renal or hepatic impairment and heart failure.

Patients treated with this drug reported a significant improvement in walking ability, speed, stair-climbing ability and calf pain severity as compared with placebo (p < 0.001).[10] Its mode of action is via vasodilatation and antiplatelet effects.

Cilostazol is contraindicated in patients with severe hepatic or renal impairment. Patients should be assessed for improvement after 3 months.

More information available at the British National Formulary website (www.bnf.org).

Patients in whom cilostazol is contraindicated, naftidrofuryl can be used as a second choice; naftidrofuryl can alleviate symptoms of IC. Patients treated with this drug should be assessed for improvement after 3–6 months.

Inositol nicotinate, pentoxifylline and cinnarizine are not established as being effective for the treatment of intermittent claudication.

More information available at the British National Formulary website (www.bnf.org).

Surgical

Immediate relief of symptoms can be provided by endovascular interventions but the cost-effectiveness and an apparent lack of durability remain a major issue.[12]

Percutaneous balloon angioplasty has been shown to be effective in improving walking distance. Patients with severe impairment of quality of life may benefit from this procedure.

Femoro-popliteal bypass is reserved for those who are not responsive to any of the above measures.

KEY POINTS

- Around 30% of patients with symptoms of IC die within 5 years because of cardiovascular disease.
- The prevalence of IC increases with age.
- GPs can play a major role in identifying patients with IC and in managing the condition.

References

1 Fowkes F, Housley E, Cawood EH, *et al.* Edinburgh Artery Study: prevalence of asymptomatic and symptomatic peripheral arterial disease in the general population. *Int J Epidemiol.* 1991: **20**(2): 384–92.

2 Caspary L, Taylor LM, Porter JM. Epidemiology of vascular disease. *Dis Manage Health Outcomes.* 1997; **2**(Suppl. 1): 9–17.

3 Stanley G. The patient with intermittent claudication. *Practitioner.* 2005; **249**(1670): 318, 320–4.

4 Dormandy J, Heeck L, Vig S. The natural history of claudication: risk to life and limb. *Semin Vasc Surg.* 1999; **12**(2): 123–37.

5 Tierney S, Fennessy F, Hayes DB. ABC of arterial and vascular disease. Secondary prevention of peripheral vascular disease. *BMJ.* 2003; **320**(7244): 1262–5.

6 Leng GC, Fowler B, Ernst E. Exercise for intermittent claudication. *Cochrane Database Syst Rev.* 2000; **2**: CD000990.

7 TASC Working Group. Management of peripheral arterial disease: TransAtlantic Inter-Society Consensus (TASC). *J Vasc Surg.* 2000; 31(Suppl.): S1–296.

8 The Heart Outcomes Prevention Evaluation Study Investigators. Effects of an angiotensin-converting-enzyme inhibitor, ramipril, on cardiovascular events in high-risk patients. *N Engl J Med.* 2000; **342**(3): 145–53.

9 Chapman TM, Goa KL. Cilostazol: a review of its use in intermittent claudication. *Am J Cardiovasc Drugs.* 2003; **3**(2): 117–38.

10 Regensteiner JG, Ware JE, McCarthy WJ *et al.* Effect of cilostazol on treadmill walking, community-based walking ability and health-related quality of life in patients with intermittent claudication due to peripheral arterial disease: meta-analysis of six randomised controlled trials. *J Am Geriatr Soc.* 2002; **50**(12): 1939–46.

11 Antithrombotic Trialists' (ATT) Collaboration. Aspirin in the primary prevention of vascular disease: collaborative meta-analysis of individual participant data from randomised trials. *Lancet.* 2009; **373**(9678): 1849–60.

12 Whyman MR, Fowkes FG, Kerracher EM. Is intermittent claudication improved by percutaneous transluminal angioplasty? A randomized controlled trial. *J Vasc Surg.* 1997; **26**(4): 551–7.

13 Williams B, Poulter NR, Brown MJ *et al.* British Hypertension Society Guidelines for management of hypertension: report of the fourth working party of the British Hypertension Society 2004-BHS 1V. *J Hum Hypertens.* 2004; 18: 139–85.

14 NICE Clinical Guideline Groups. Hypertension: management of hypertension in adults in primary care. *NICE* CG 34, June 2006.

9

Leg ulcers

Adele Marie Scimone

It is widely published that chronic ulceration of the leg affects 1%–2% of the population and the majority of this ulceration occurs in people aged 65 or over, although this is not always the case.[1] Under the age of 40 the prevalence of ulceration in men and women is similar but with increasing age it is higher in women.

A leg ulcer may be defined as 'A loss of skin below the knee which takes more than 6 weeks to heal'[2] and can be classified according to aetiology. In the United Kingdom approximately 70% of ulcers are primarily caused by chronic venous hypertension, which is the insufficient return of venous blood from the lower limb and is manifested by pathological changes in the skin and subcutaneous tissue.

Poor arterial blood supply accounts for 10%. A further 10% have both venous and arterial pathology and are known as mixed ulcers. The remaining 10% are made up of diabetic ulceration, which usually occurs on the foot and from other causes.[3]

Other causes of leg ulceration include pyoderma gangrenosum, vasculitic, tropical and malignant ulcerations and it is important to be familiar with these.[4]

It is estimated that chronic wounds costs the National Health Service (NHS) 2.3 to 3.1 billion per year[5] and the ulcers are mostly managed in the community by district nurses who are highly skilled and trained in their management, and who refer on to specialists such as tissue viability nurses or vascular surgeons as necessary.

Leg ulcers seriously impact on a patient's quality of life, causing pain, social isolation and embarrassment.[6] Identifying the underlying pathology of the leg ulcer is extremely important in planning appropriate management and requires a full holistic assessment of the patient, the limb and the ulcer.

Assessment

The assessment should include a full history of the ulceration, any previous ulceration and time to healing and treatments used. Medical and surgical history should be obtained – paying particular attention to pathologies that would predispose to venous disease and those to arterial disease (*see* Table 9.1) and these diseases should be specifically asked about, as should diabetes, which is a significant risk factor for peripheral vascular disease. Patients with rheumatoid arthritis/connective tissue disease may develop vasculitis, which causes occlusion of the small vessels leading to tissue ischaemia[7] so it is useful to have this information to aid in diagnosis. By obtaining this medical history from a patient, the examiner is attempting to identify risk factors, disease states and vascular history commonly associated with arterial, venous or comorbid (non-vascular) pathology. Patients with mixed ulcers may present with a combination of the features described in Table 9.1.

TABLE 9.1 Venous disease and arterial disease: pathologies

ARTERIAL	VENOUS
Hypertension	Past history of DVT/phlebitis
Coronary artery disease/peripheral vascular disease	Recent orthopaedic surgery
Diabetes mellitus	Recent pelvic surgery
Rheumatoid arthritis	Leg trauma
Transient ischaemic attacks/CVA	Varicose veins
Family history CV disease	Previous vein stripping
Age	Family history of venous ulceration
Cigarette smoking	Multiple pregnancies
High cholesterol	Occupation involving long period of standing
Hypertension	Raised intra-abdominal pressure
Arterial disease elsewhere	Previous fractures

Source: Royal College of Nursing[8]

Social and environmental contributing factors such as smoking and obesity should be assessed. Information on occupation, both past and present, should be gained as occupations that involve prolonged standing – particularly in warm conditions – could contribute to venous pathology. Medications both prescribed and over-the-counter should be reviewed for their effect on wound healing and a knowledge of medication is essential as some can actually cause ulceration.[9] In addition, any complementary therapies that the patient may be using on the skin or wound, or taking internally, should be documented in the notes.

Family history is also important, as arterial and venous disease tend to have familial links.[8] Patience on the part of the examiner is essential as is the ability to actively listen to the patient in order to elicit information.

Many leg ulcer services have a comprehensive leg ulcer assessment form, which assists in gathering this information.

Physical assessment should include blood pressure, pulse and urinalysis to form a baseline and detect any underlying abnormality such as diabetes, hypertension or arrhythmias.

Assessment of the patient's clinical signs and symptoms should be carried out (*see* Table 9.3) and both limbs examined for venous and/or arterial disease.

TABLE 9.2 Signs of arterial and venous disease

SIGNS OF ARTERIAL DISEASE	SIGNS OF VENOUS DISEASE
Ulcers with a 'punched out' appearance with base of wound poorly perfused and pale.[8] *See* Figures 9.1 and 9.2.	Usually shallow ulcers – situated on the gaiter area of the leg.[8] *See* Figure 9.3.
Cold, shiny, pale, hairless skin and thickened nails[8]	Varicose eczema (dermatitis)[8]
Limb is red/dusky blue/pink on dependency and turns pale on elevation[8]	Pigmentation[8]
Gangrenous toes[8]	Telangiectasia or ankle flare[8]
Absent pedal pulses[10]	Lipodermatosclerosis[8]
Poor capillary refilling time[9]	Atrophie blanche[8]
Localised oedema[10]	Oedema[8]
Pain in limb relieved by positioning leg in a dependent position[8]	Varicose veins[8]

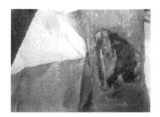

FIGURE 9.1 Arterial ulcer

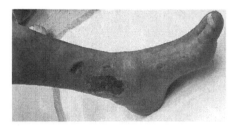

FIGURE 9.2 Mixed ulcer

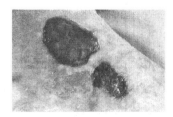

FIGURE 9.3 Venous ulcer

The patient should also be asked if they have any pain, which should be assessed for severity and type – what exacerbates it or relieves it as this may give information as to the type of ulcer, for instance arterial disease may be responsible for pain which may be aggravated by limb elevation or exercise. Pain on walking could indicate claudication, which is seen in moderate stenosis and occlusive states and presents as intermittent pain associated with exercise. This condition is due to the inability of the collateral circulation to meet the needs of the exercising muscle.[11] A sudden increase in pain may indicate infection or advancement of any peripheral vascular disease and reassessment of the arterial status should be carried out.[8]

The wound itself should be examined, as should the surrounding skin. The site of the ulcer should be recorded and measurements taken; these should be repeated at least monthly to monitor healing and evaluate if the treatment plan is working. The local wound environment should be optimised. The TIME Framework is a simple but useful tool: Tissue, Infection/inflammation, Moisture/exudate levels, Epithelial edge advancement, which aids wound bed preparation and focuses the practitioner on the condition of the wound bed.[12] The peri-wound area should be assessed for signs of erythema or maceration. Any suspicious or non-healing ulcer should be referred for biopsy to exclude malignancy.

The skin should be inspected for signs of venous insufficiency such as eczema, lipodermatosclerosis (fibrosis of the skin and subcutaneous tissue), pigmentation, atrophie blanch, ankle flare and the presence of varicose veins or for signs of arterial insufficiency such as thickened toenails, shiny hairless skin, pallor and sluggish capillary refill among others. Oedema may occur in both arterial and venous disease. The clinician should enquire about previous topical treatments. Patients with venous disease are very susceptible to irritant and allergic reactions.

Ankle movement should be examined as limited ankle movement can interfere with the action of the calf muscle pump.

Further investigations such as full blood count, urea and electrolytes, liver function tests, lipid profile and inflammatory markers may be required to identify any underlying factors that are contributing to non-healing, but these should not be needed routinely. If rheumatoid arthritis or other connective tissue disorder is suspected then an autoimmune screen should also be carried out.[9] A nutritional assessment should be undertaken in all patients presenting with an ulcer. Obesity may lead to reduced mobility and puts excessive strain on the limb while malnutrition contributes to poor healing.[8]

All patients presenting with an ulcer should be screened for arterial disease by measurement of the Ankle Brachial Pressure Index (ABPI) using the handheld Doppler and by staff who are trained to undertake this measurement.[8] The Doppler assessment of the lower limb seeks to determine the resting pressure index, i.e. comparing the resting brachial systolic pressure to the resting ankle systolic pressure, and this is presented as a ratio. The ABPI is meaningless when used in isolation and should form part of the full holistic assessment; it is an indicator of suitability for compression therapy or the need for patient referral for vascular consultation.[13] A normal ABPI does not diagnose a venous ulcer but forms part of the clinical picture.

The procedure for carrying out an ABPI is widely reported in the literature[14–16] and is summarised with interpretation of the results in Box 9.1 and Table 9.3.

The figure 0.8 is given as the cut-off point for high compression therapy, yet evidence to support this is lacking.[17] We should not rely on a single ratio as this does not take into account the different perfusion pressures between the three vessels at the ankle. A difference of 15 mmHg or greater indicates a proximal stenosis or occlusion in the vessel with the lower pressure.[18] Such a pressure difference will increase the risk of pressure damage to the related zone of the calf, irrespective of the ABPI.[14] Therefore, looking at the pressure differences between vessels and listening to the quality of the audible signals is imperative.

Artificially high readings may be obtained in patients with diabetes, renal disease and oedema due to non-compressible arteries.[19] If any doubt exists then further investigations such as Doppler waveform analysis or toe pressures should be performed. If the arterial status cannot be ascertained then a vascular referral should be made for further investigations.

The healthy artery produces three phases and is known as triphasic (see Figure 9.4). This is an initial forward flow, rising to a peak at the peak of systole, a reverse flow during diastole and finally a further forward flow during diastole. The last two reflect the elastic recoil of the vessel.[20]

As the vessel walls lose some of their elasticity due to age and early atherosclerosis it produces a two-phase or biphasic signal where the reverse flow component is lost. As disease progresses a monophasic signal, which gives only one sound of a much lower frequency, can be heard representing a single forward flow through a stenosed or rigid vessel (*see* Figure 9.5).[20] These can be presented as an audible signal or from a visual waveform.

If signal quality is poor with monophasic signals then referral to a vascular specialist is required.[14] Many patients with peripheral vascular disease will be treated conservatively but it is important that this decision is made by a vascular surgeon along with the patient. As peripheral vascular disease is an indicator of the general state of the arteries, patients with this disease are at risk of mortality from cardiovascular causes.[21] It is therefore essential that the patient's general practitioner be notified in order that appropriate medical management be commenced and the patient advised on risk factor modification.

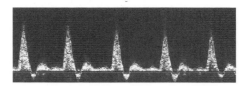

FIGURE 9.4 Triphasic waveform

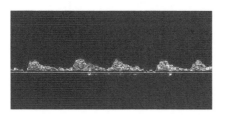

FIGURE 9.5 Monophasic waveform

Procedure for carrying out an ABPI

Ensure correct probe size is used – an 8 mHz probe for general use or a 5 mHz probe for oedematous limbs. Clean the probe with an alcohol swab prior to use.

BOX 9.1 ABPI PROCEDURE

1 Explain procedure and allow patient to ask questions.

2 Ensure patient is positioned comfortably with trousers, shoes and socks removed, with consideration being given to privacy and dignity.

3 Wash hands.

4 Position patient in supine position on the examination couch and leave to rest for 15 minutes.

5 Remove ulcer dressings and cover wounds with a light non-adherent dressing or cling film.

6 **Measure the brachial systolic pressure:**
   - place an appropriate-sized cuff around the upper arm and locate the brachial pulse, applying ultrasound gel over the pulse
   - angle the Doppler probe at a 45 degree angle toward the heart and move until the best signal is heard – avoid excessive pressure over the artery
   - inflate blood pressure cuff 20–30 mmHg beyond the point at which the last arterial signal was detected, then deflate the cuff slowly and record the pressure at which the signal returns
   - repeat the procedure for the other arm.
   - Use the highest of the two readings for the ABPI.

7 **Measure the ankle systolic pressure:**
   - place an appropriate-sized cuff around the ankle immediately above the malleoli
   - locate the dorsalis pedis or anterior tibial artery, apply ultrasound gel and continue as for brachial pressure, recording the pressure in the same way
   - repeat the procedure for the posterior tibial artery
   - use the highest of the readings to calculate the ABPI
   - repeat for the other leg.

   - $$ABPI = \frac{\text{Highest ankle pressure for that leg}}{\text{Highest of brachial pressures for each arm}}$$

   - Inaccuracies may occur when:

- a standardised procedure is not followed[22]
- the blood pressure cuff is not placed correctly at the ankle[23]
- the cuff-size selection is incorrect[23]
- the patient is not rested prior to testing[24]
- gross oedema is present.[25]

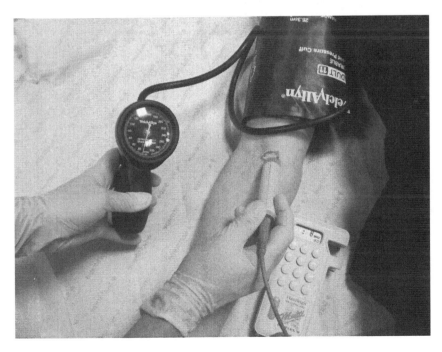

FIGURE 9.6A Obtaining the brachial systolic pressure

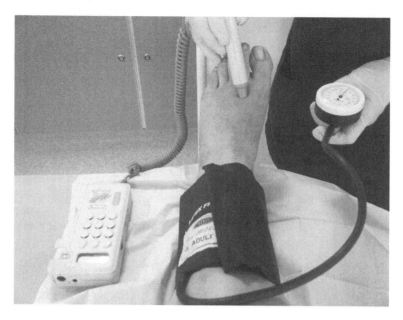

FIGURE 9.6B Obtaining the dorsalis pedis systolic pressure

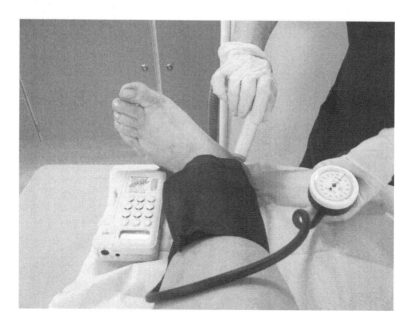

FIGURE 9.6C Obtaining the posterior tibial systolic pressure

Interpretation of ABPI (subject to local protocols)

TABLE 9.3 Interpretation of ABPI

> 1.3	Indicates a falsely elevated reading which could be due to vessel calcification or oedema	Further investigations required
1 - 1.3	Indicates normal arterial flow	
< 0.9	Mild degree of arterial involvement	High compression therapy may be used after consideration of other factors, i.e. diabetes.
0.8	Indicates there is 80% blood flow to the foot	Recognised as the cut off point for high compression therapy
< 0.8	Moderate arterial impairment	Refer to Vascular Surgeon if present with one or more of the following symptoms: ischaemic rest pain, intermittent claudication, worsening ulceration, ischaemic changes to feet or toes
0.6 – 0.8	Indicates a level of arterial disease where reduced compression may be used under strict supervision	Refer to Tissue Viability/Vascular nursing team
< 0.5	Indicates severe arterial impairment	Urgent referral to Vascular Surgeon. Do not use compression therapy

Source: Oldham Community Health Services 2008 (Local Protocol)[26]

Toe pressures

When an ABPI is inconclusive due to there being no cut-off point – possibly due to oedema or due to calcification of the vessel wall – toe pressures may be carried out. Toe pressures test the flow of blood through the big toe where the vessels are less likely to be calcified.[27] They are also useful when placing the cuff over an ulcer at the ankle would cause pain to the patient.

Toe pressures, however, are subject to significant positional and temperature variation,[19] which can make this procedure more difficult to carry out. The investigation can be carried out using a Doppler probe but is more accurate using strain gauge or photoplethysmography.[28]

As the ABPI may change over time it is important that this test is repeated, particularly if any deterioration in the ulcer occurs or at 3-monthly intervals;[8] however, this is often subject to individual trust protocols or practitioners.

Compression therapy

It is well documented that the cornerstone of treatment and prevention for venous ulceration is graduated compression therapy.[5] The situation becomes far more complex when there is concomitant peripheral vascular disease. As a high proportion of leg ulcers occur in the older people, many of these patients will have some degree of atherosclerosis – often without symptoms. This is particularly true if the disease is not yet severe and the individual has limited mobility so that intermittent claudication during walking is not a feature – this is often an early symptom in mobile patients. Hence why it is vital that the vascular status of the limb is ascertained prior to commencing any treatment with compression therapy. Where there is peripheral vascular disease, the balance has to be found whereby the venous component is treated to best effect by reduction of the underlying venous hypertension without further compromise of the arterial circulation.

Compression therapy is the application of a pressure gradient that helps counteract the effects of venous hypertension – improving venous return.[13] Providing the level of compression does not impede arterial flow the effects can be quite dramatic, reducing oedema and pain and promoting healing and prevention of ulcers caused by venous insufficiency.[29] Treatment will depend upon the severity of the arterial component. In patients with an ABPI of 0.8 or above high compression therapy is generally considered safe, providing all other factors have been considered.[30]

The sub-bandage pressure is based on Laplace's equation, which, put

simply, is the result of the tension induced in the bandage during application, the number of layers used, the width of the bandage and the limb
circumference (*see* Box 9.2).[31] Therefore, sub-bandage pressure is directly
proportional to the bandage tension, but inversely proportional to limb
circumference. Many authors advocate the use of 40 mmHg sub-bandage
pressure at the ankle reducing to approximately 20 mmHg at the knee.[32,33]
At present there is no international consensus of optimal sub-bandage pressures with much higher values being used successfully across Europe[34] both
in bandage and hosiery pressures. However, patient factors are an important
component in any treatment's success and patients may not tolerate pressures that are very high.[32]

BOX 9.2 THE LAPLACE EQUATION

$$\text{Pressure} = \frac{\text{Tension of bandage} \times \text{number of layers} \times \text{constant}}{\text{Circumference of limb} \times \text{width of bandage}}$$

There are several systems of applying this level of compression and it is
important that the patient makes an informed choice in deciding which
system to use as this will aid healing and concordance.[35] Concordance with
compression therapy may be better achieved by listening to the patient's
perceptions and finding the most acceptable way of applying the highest
recommended pressures that can be tolerated. An understanding by nurses
of how compression works and the underlying pathophysiology of venous
hypertension would allow greater creativity when selecting the appropriate system for the patient and to aid concordance by helping the patient
understand their condition.

Bandages are classified according to the compression they provide when
applied in a certain manner and also as to whether they are elastic or
inelastic.

Four-layer bandaging was developed in the mid 1980s[13] and consists of
wool padding, a type 2 crepe bandage, a type 3a light compression bandage
(applied in a figure-eight configuration) and a cohesive type 3b compression
bandage (applied in a spiral); combined, they effectively give 40 mmHg at
the ankle, reducing to approximately 20 mmHg at the knee.[36] This is based

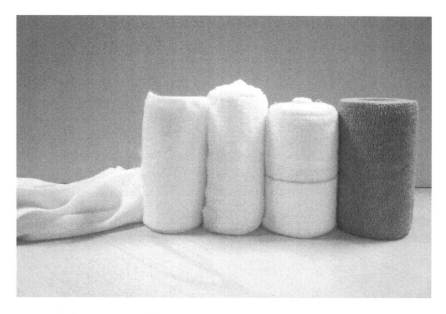

FIGURE 9.7 Components of the four-layer system

on an ankle circumference of between 18 cm and 25 cm and the limb must be measured regularly to ensure the correct system is used. Modified systems are used for limb sizes outside this range. Cotton tubular bandage is placed next to the skin to prevent any irritation from the padding layer.

In order to achieve graduated compression the limb shape must be taken into consideration and padding applied to achieve a graduated increase up the leg. This is particularly important in limbs with muscle loss over the calf and the 'inverted champagne bottle' leg.[37]

These elastic bandages give sustained compression during both mobilisation and resting and are effective for up to 1 week. They are applied in a 50% overlap with 50% extension. *See* Figures 9.8a–f for application.

Short stretch bandages are inelastic and provide a rigid case around the limb that the calf muscle works against during mobilisation – assisting in venous return. They are applied at full stretch with 50% overlap in a spiral fashion. Again, padding must be used to protect bony prominences, tendons and to shape the limb. Short-term bandages can be useful in reducing oedema but, due to their inelastic nature, do not follow the limb as oedema reduces and therefore may need to be changed frequently to prevent slippage in the initial phase. These bandages are not as bulky as the four-layer system

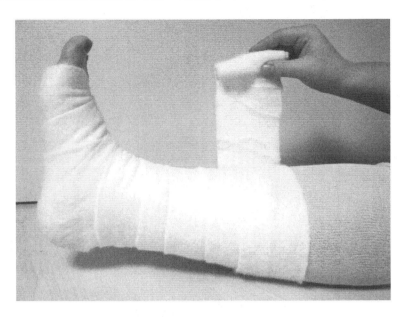

FIGURE 9.8A Application of the padding layer

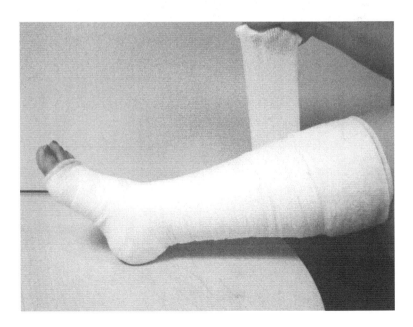

FIGURE 9.8B Type 2a bandage applied in a spiral

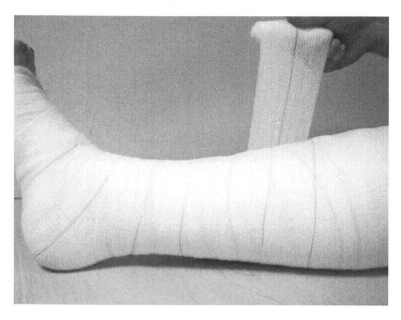

FIGURE 9.8C Type 3a bandage applied at 50% stretch, 50% overlap in a figure of eight

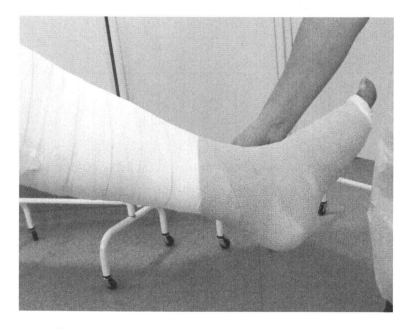

FIGURE 9.8D Type 3b bandage applied at 50% stretch, 50% overlap in a spiral

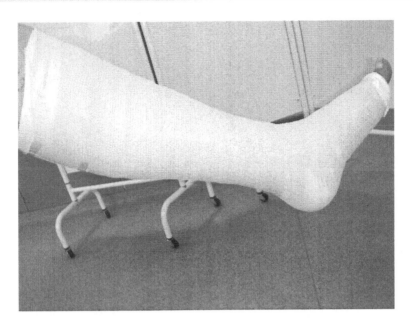

FIGURE 9.8E Completed four-layer bandage

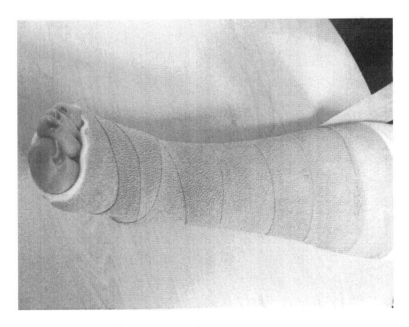

FIGURE 9.8F Completed four-layer bandage

so may be more suitable for patients wishing to wear their own footwear. They are not suitable for immobile patients as they require the use of the foot and calf muscle pump in order to be effective. Due to their stiffness they provide high working and low resting pressures.[38]

Recent studies have shown the effectiveness of the newer multilayer hosiery kits that provide high compression of 40 mmHg at the ankle.[39] These may be of benefit for patients with non-complex wounds with low exudates – particularly those who wish to self-manage, participate in their own care or wear their own footwear. However, the patient must be chosen carefully as this option may not be suitable for fragile skin or where there are other skin problems.[40] There are also some two-layer bandage kits now available that may be suitable as an alternative in some patients. Sub-bandage pressures are affected by many factors including the application technique and the skill of the bandager. Some bandage manufacturers have attempted to overcome this by adding visual aids to the bandage to help achieve the correct tension.

It is important prior to the application of compression therapy to observe for the presence of neuropathy as pressure damage may not be felt, due to the lack of normal pain responses.[41] Cardiac failure must also be considered as the application of high compression therapy increases the pre-load of the heart by around 5% due to the fluid shift into the circulation.[30]

Time to healing for a venous ulcer will depend upon the size of the ulcer and the length of time the patient has had the ulcer prior to treatment.[42] By predicting healing times early on, treatment may be optimised and any increased expenditure associated with more advanced therapies may be offset by an overall reduction in costs due to faster healing and improved quality of life.

Reduced compression therapy may be used in patients who have an ABPI < 0.8 but it is important that this is closely supervised and performed under the guidance of the tissue viability or vascular nurse specialist. Reduced compression may be achieved by omitting the type 3a light compression bandage, giving approximately 23 mmHg at the ankle, or by omitting the final cohesive bandage, which will achieve around 17 mmHg at the ankle. In my trust a reduced compression of 10–12 mmHg is used for some by applying the type 3a light compression bandage in a simple spiral rather than a figure of eight and omitting the cohesive type 3b bandage. The exact level of reduced compression will depend upon the severity of symptoms and the patient's ability to tolerate it.[43]

Prevention of recurrence

Ulcer recurrence rates have been shown to be as high as 26%–29%.[44] Research is currently focused on the role of superficial venous surgery.[38] Duplex ultrasound studies have shown that 50% of venous ulcers may simply be the result of superficial reflux and as such may respond to surgery.[45]

Adding these investigations would have initial cost implications, however, although the studies to date have shown that recurrence rates are greatly reduced following superficial venous surgery, with potential cost savings in the long term;[46] It would appear that surgery does have a preventative role to play.

Hosiery is currently the mainstay of treatment for prevention of recurrence. However, very few trials have evaluated its effectiveness.[47] A Cochrane review concluded that there was no current evidence that high compression was more effective that moderate compression in prevention of recurrence and that concordance is lower in patients wearing high compression hosiery. Patients should be prescribed the highest level of compression stocking that they are able to tolerate.[47]

It is important that the skin is kept hydrated, as dry, rough skin is more prone to damage than supple, moisturised skin. Daily use of a simple moisturiser and avoidance of soap will help to prevent abrasions that could lead to ulceration.

Accurate measurement of the limb should ensure that the hosiery is a good fit. If stockings are too long they can roll down, causing a harmful tourniquet effect. If too short they can cause a band of oedema above the stocking. If necessary, hosiery can be made to measure. The ABPI should be carried out each time compression hosiery is prescribed – although this is subject to local protocols, current guidelines suggest every 6 months.[8]

KEY POINTS

- Approximately 70% of leg ulcers are venous.
- Full holistic assessment is the key to management.
- All patients presenting with an ulcer must be screened for arterial disease by measurement of the ABPI.
- Compression therapy is the mainstay of treatment for venous ulceration.

> • When complicated by concomitant peripheral vascular disease, the venous component must be treated without further compromise of the arterial circulation.

References

1 Briggs M, Closs SJ. The prevalence of leg ulceration: a review of the literature. *EWMA Journal.* 2003; **3**(2): 14–20.

2 Dale J, Callam M, Ruckley C *et al.* Chronic ulcers of the leg: a study of prevalence in a Scottish community. *Health Bull (Edinb).* 1983; **41**(6): 310–14.

3 Nelzen O, Berquist D, Lindhagen A. Leg ulcer aetiology: a cross-sectional population study. *J Vasc Surg.* 1991; **14**(4): 557–64.

4 Moffatt C, Martin R, Smithdale R. *Leg Ulcer Management.* Oxford: Blackwell; 2007.

5 Simon DA, Dix FP, McCollum CN. Management of venous leg ulcers. *BMJ.* 2004; **328**(7452); 1358–62.

6 Chase SK, Savage A, Melloni H. A forever healing: the lived experience of venous ulcer disease. *J Vasc Nurs.* 1997; **15**(2): 73–8.

7 Clinical Resource Efficiency Support Team (CREST). *Guidelines for the Assessment and Management of Leg Ulceration.* Northern Ireland: CREST; 1998.

8 Royal College of Nursing (RCN). *Clinical Guidelines for the Management of Patients with Venous Leg Ulcers.* London: RCN; 2006.

9 Nelzen OP. Venous ulcers patient assessment. In: Morrison M, Moffatt CJ, Franks P, editors. *Leg Ulcers: a problem-based learning approach.* London: Mosby; 2007, pp. 155–67.

10 Clarke-Moloney M, Grace P. Understanding the underlying causes of chronic leg ulceration. *J Wound Care.* 2004; **13**(6): 215–18.

11 Baun J. Practical arterial evaluation of the lower extremity. *Journal of Diagnostic Medical Sonography.* 2004; **20**(1): 5–13.

12 Falanga V. Wound bed preparation: science applied to practice. In: *European Wound Management Association (EWMA) Position Document: wound bed preparation in practice.* London: MEP Ltd; 2004, pp. 2–5.

13 Moffatt CJ. *Compression Therapy in Practice.* Aberdeen: Wounds UK; 2007.

14 Vowden KR, Goulding V, Vowden P. Hand-held Doppler assessment for peripheral arterial disease. *J Wound Care.* 1996; **5**(3): 125–8.

15 Ruff D. Doppler assessment: calculating an ankle brachial pressure index. *Nurs Times.* 2003; **99**(42): 62–5.

16 Stubbing NJ, Bailey P, Poole M. Protocol for accurate assessment of ABPI in patients with leg ulcers. *J Wound Care*. 1997; **6**(9): 417–18.

17 Vowden K, Vowden P. Doppler and the ABPI: how good is our understanding? *J Wound Care*. 2001; **10**(6): 199–202.

18 Sumner DS. Non-invasive assessment of peripheral arterial occlusive disease. In: Rutherford KS, editor. *Vascular Surgery*. 3rd ed. Philadelphia: WB Saunders; 1998, pp. 41–60.

19 Carter SA. Role of pressure measurement. In: Bernstein ER, editor. *Vascular Diagnosis*. St Louis: Mosby; 1993, pp. 486–512.

20 Baker N, Rayman G. Clinical evaluation of Doppler signals. *Diabetic Foot Journal*. 1999; **2**(1): S22–25.

21 Parker D. Peripheral arterial disease. *Ind Nurs*. 2009 (Sept): 39–40.

22 Jeelani NUO, Braithwaite BD, Tomlin C *et al*. Variation of method for measurement of brachial artery pressure significantly affects Ankle Brachial Pressure Index values. *Eur J Vasc Endovasc Surg*. 2000; **20**(1): 25–8.

23 Bonham PA. Get the LEAD out: non-invasive assessment of lower extremity arterial disease using ankle brachial index and toe brachial index measurements. *J Wound Ostomy Continence*. 2006; **33**(1): 30–41.

24 Vowden KR, Goulding V, Vowden P. Hand-held Doppler assessment for peripheral arterial disease. *J Wound Care*. 1996; **5**(3): 125–8.

25 Moffatt C, O'Hare P. Ankle pulses are not sufficient to detect impaired arterial circulation in patients with leg ulcers. *J Wound Care*. 1995; **4**(2); 134–8.

26 Oldham Community Health Services (OCHS). *Guidelines for the Management of Leg Ulcers*. Oldham: OCHS; 2009.

27 Vowden P. Doppler ultrasound in the management of the diabetic foot. *Diabetic Foot Journal*. 1999; **2**(1): S16–7.

28 Sumner DS. Mercury strain-gauge plethysmography. In: Bernstein ER, editor. *Vascular Diagnosis*. St Louis: Mosby; 1993, pp. 205–33.

29 Partsch H. Understanding the physiological effects of compression. In: *European Wound Management Association (EWMA) Position Document: understanding compression therapy*. London: MEP Ltd; 2003, p. 2.

30 Marston W, Vowden K. Compression therapy: a guide to safe practice. In: *European Wound Management Association (EWMA) Position Document: understanding compression therapy*. London: MEP Ltd; 2003, p. 11.

31 Thomas S. The use of the Laplace equation in the calculation of sub-bandage pressure. *EWMA Journal*. 2003; **3**(1): 21–3.

32 Moore Z. Compression bandaging: are practitioners achieving the ideal sub-bandage pressures? *J Wound Care.* 2002; **11**(7): 265–8.

33 Sieggreen MY, Kline RA. Recognizing and Managing Venous Leg Ulcers. *Adv Skin Wound Care.* 2004; **17**(6): 311–13.

34 Clark M. Compression bandages: principles and definitions. In: *European Wound Management Association (EWMA) Position Document: understanding compression therapy.* London: MEP Ltd; 2003, p. 5.

35 Moffatt CJ. Factors that affect concordance. *J Wound Care.* 2004; **13**(7): 291–4.

36 Moffatt CJ. *Four-Layer Bandaging: from concept to practice. Part 1: the development of the four-layer system.* Available at: www.worldwidewounds.com/2004/december/Moffatt/Developing-Four-Layer-Bandaging.html (accessed 15 December 2009).

37 World Union Wound Healing Societies. *Compression in Venous Leg Ulcers: a consensus document.* London: MEP Ltd; 2008.

38 Rajendran S, Rigby AJ, Anans SC. Venous leg ulcer treatment and practice – part 3: the use of compression therapy systems. *J Wound Care.* 2007; **16**(3): 107–9.

39 Cullum N, Nelson EA, Fletcher AW *et al.* Compression for venous leg ulcers. *Cochrane Database Syst Rev.* 2001; **2**: CD000265. DOI: 10.1002/14651858. CD000265.

40 Cullum N, Fletcher A, Semlyen A *et al.* Compression therapy for venous leg ulcers. *Qual Health Care.* 1997; **6**(4): 226–31.

41 Marston W, Vowden K. Compression therapy: a guide to safe practice. In: *European Wound Management Association (EWMA) Position Document: understanding compression therapy.* London: MEP Ltd; 2003, p. 11.

42 Margolis DJ, Berlin JA, Strom BI. A simple model based on wound size and duration predicted healing of venous leg ulcers at 24 weeks. *Evid Based Med.* 2001; **24**(2): 36–8.

43 Moffatt C, Harper P. *Leg Ulcers: access to clinical education.* London: Churchill Livingstone; 1997.

44 Franks PJ, Oldroyd MI, Dickson D *et al.* Risk factors for leg ulcer recurrence: a randomized trial of two types of compression stocking. *Age Ageing.* 1995; **24**(6): 490–4.

45 Vowden K. How good are we at preventing venous leg ulceration? *Leg Ulcer Forum Journal.* 2005; **19**: 29–32.

46 Gohel MS, Barwell JR, Taylor M *et al.* Long term results of compression therapy

alone versus compression therapy plus surgery in chronic venous ulceration (ESCHAR): randomised controlled trial. *BMJ*. 2007; **335**(7610): 55–6.

47 Nelson EA, Bell-Syer SEM, Cullum NA. Compression for preventing recurrence of venous ulcers. *Cochrane Database Syst Rev*. 2000; **4**: CD002303. DOI.10.1002/14651858.CD002303.

10

Ankle Brachial Pressure Index

The Ankle Brachial Pressure Index compares the blood pressure in the leg arteries with that in the brachial artery using Doppler to detect the flow of blood and sphygmomanometer to measure the pressure. Dividing the highest pressure at which the Doppler pulsation was detected in the ankle by the highest brachial artery pressure gives a value of ABPI. Ankle Brachial Pressure Index (ABPI) is easy to measure and can be measured in a primary care setting by a trained practice nurse or a general practitioner.

It is a simple, relatively inexpensive and accurate test and has become the mainstay of confirmation in diagnosis of peripheral arterial disease (PAD). Findings from clinical examination have poor sensitivity in confirmation of diagnosis in symptomatic PAD patients. It predicts angiography results more accurately than is possible using history and clinical examination.[1] Angiography in lower extremity is reserved for those with advanced disease in whom surgical intervention is being considered.[1]

It has been reported to have a sensitivity ranging from 79%–95% with a specificity consistently > 95% in patients in whom there is a suspicion of PAD.[1]

Equipment

The equipment needed to perform an ABPI is:
- a handheld Doppler with a probe (an 8 MHz probe is ideal for ABPI on

average-sized limbs; a 5 MHz is ideal for oedematous limbs; to assess arterial and venous blood flow a frequency of 5–8 MHz is required)
- ultrasound gel
- tissues
- cling film if there is an ulcer to cover
- an aneroid sphygmomanometer – electronic sphygmomanometer must not be used.

Cost
An Ankle Brachial Pressure Index kit can cost between £800 and £900.

Patient preparation, procedure and interpretation of result

(Also *see* Chapter 9, Leg ulcers.) In a normal person the pressure at the ankle is slightly greater than at the elbow. An ABPI value greater than 0.9 is considered normal.

An ABPI of greater than 1.3 suggests calcification of the arteries, which in turn suggests severe peripheral vascular disease. Compression bandaging should not be applied for these patients.

An ABPI between 1 and 1.2 indicates normal blood flow and is safe for compression.

An ABPI of 0.9 indicates mild obstruction and is safe for compression.

An ABPI of 0.8 is the lowest level at which compression can be safely applied.

All patients with an ABPI of less than 0.8 should be referred for vascular assessment.

A value of 0.6 and below indicates severe peripheral vascular disease requiring urgent assessment by a vascular surgeon.

Failure to identify arterial signals at the ankle requires an opinion from a vascular specialist. In atrial fibrillation it may be difficult to measure the systolic pressure because of irregular pulse. Leaving the cuff inflated for a long period of time can cause the ankle pressure reading to fall by producing a hyperaemic response.[2–4]

ABPI does not assess the micro-vessel disease and has its limitations in diabetes, rheumatoid arthritis and vasculitis.

It is inversely related to blood pressure,[4] therefore the ABPI reading may be low in patients with hypotension.

An artificially high reading may be obtained in the following:

- diabetics, due to calcification of arteries
- patients with gross oedema
- renal disease patients.

ABPI should only be interpreted alongside clinical examination.

Repeat Doppler

Patients should have a repeat Doppler at 3-monthly intervals, or sooner[5] if they experience:

- deterioration of leg ulcer
- worsening of night pain
- inability to comply with compression
- claudication.

TABLE 10.1 Venous or arterial disease

VENOUS	ARTERIAL
Pain when the leg is dependent, relieved by elevation	Rest pain, worse on night Patient hangs the limb out of bed
Haemosiderin staining Oedema Woody, scaly skin	Loss of colour on elevation Atrophic shiny skin
ABPI 0.8–1.2	ABPI < 0.6
Venous ulcer is shallow irregular shape	Arterial ulcer is deeper punched out edge Sloughy, necrotic tissue
Ulcer above the malleolus on the lower third of calf	Ulcer on the toes or foot
Varicose veins	No varicose veins
Varicose eczema	No varicose eczema

Training

The Doppler must be undertaken by a professional – a nurse or general practitioner who is clinically competent and confident. All practitioners must receive adequate training and supervision before using the Doppler.[2,6,7] The training can be obtained by attending a leg ulcer clinic or a leg ulcer management course – the professional must be supervised initially by an experienced colleague.

Decontamination

Infection control policy for the decontamination of reusable medical devices for cleaning the cuff and the Doppler probe must be observed at all times. The probe should be cleaned with pre-impregnated detergent wipes and dried with a disposable cloth. Alcohol wipes can be used if disinfection is required.

Disadvantages of the ABPI

- Performing the ABPI is time-consuming.[8]
- It is unreliable on patients with calcification of arteries.[9]
- Stiff arteries produce falsely high ankle pressure, giving a false negative.[10] This is often seen in diabetics (41% of PAD patients have diabetes).[11]
- Resting ABPI is insensitive to mild PAD.[12]
- A skilled person is needed to perform the test for accurate and consistent results.[13]

Indications of doing Doppler studies

- A high-risk indicator of PAD such as:
  — diabetes
  — smoking
  — coronary artery disease
  — hypertension
  — strong family history
  — cerebrovascular disease.
- A history of exercise-induced leg pain.
- Leg ulcer.
- Before applying compression bandaging.

Contraindications

The only absolute contraindications of measuring Ankle Brachial Pressure Index are:

- critical limb ischaemia
- deep-vein thrombosis (recent or within the last 6 weeks as it may be painful and dislodge the clot – the presence or absence of DVT must be confirmed by appropriate investigations)[14]
- cellulitis.

ABPI predictor of cardiovascular events

Ankle Brachial Pressure Index is a good predictor of subsequent cardiovascular events and death. A larger international registry of patients found that 5.4% of patients with established PAD had a major cardiovascular event at one year and 21% experienced these endpoints or hospitalization for atherosclerotic events.[15]

Eleven years follow up in the Cardiovascular Health Study found, after controlling for other risk factors, an almost two-fold increased risk for mortality in participants with ABPI 0.71 to 0.8 and 0.81 to 0.9, compared to those with ABPI 1.1 to 1.2.[16]

This test can be included in the routine screening of all hypertensives, diabetics and patients with coronary artery disease. Patients with low ABPI might benefit from addition of aspirin and statin.[17]

KEY POINTS

- ABPI is a simple diagnostic tool for the assessment of PAD.
- It can be used to evaluate the risk of overall cardiovascular morbidity.
- An ABPI < 0.9 confirms the diagnosis of PAD.
- All patients with an ABPI < 0.8 should be referred to a vascular specialist.
- Only professionals who have received specific training should perform the test.
- ABPI is not used to diagnose the type of ulcer (arterial/venous). It should be used in conjunction with medical history, examination and clinical examination of the ulcer.

References

1 Hirsch AT, Haskal ZJ, Hertzer NR *et al.* ACC/AHA 2005 Practice Guidelines for the management of patients with peripheral arterial disease (lower extremity, renal, mesenteric and abdominal aorta): a collaborative report from the American Association for Vascular Surgery, Society for Cardiovascular Angiography and Interventions, Society for Vascular Medicine and the ACC/AHA Task Force on Practice Guidelines. National Heart, Lung and Blood Institute: Society for Vascular Nursing, TransAtlantic Inter-Society Consensus and Vascular Disease Foundation, Circulation 2006; 113: e463.

2 Vowden P, Vowden K. Doppler assessment and ABPI. Interpretation in the management of leg ulceration. World Wide Wounds; 18 May 2001. www.worldwidewounds.com/2001/march/Vowden/Doppler-assessment-and-ABPI.html (accessed 10 March 2011).

3 Davies C. Use of Doppler ultrasound in leg ulcer assessment. *Nurs Stand.* 2001; **15**(44): 72–4.

4 Carser DG. Do we need to reappraise our method of interpreting the ankle brachial pressure index? *J Wound Care.* 2001; **10**(3): 59–62 (Mar 2001).

5 Simon DA, Freak L, Williams I *et al.* Progression of arterial disease in patients with healed venous ulcers. *J Wound Care.* 1994; **3**(4): 179–80.

6 Hislop C. Leg ulcer assessment by Doppler ultrasound. *Nurs Stand.* 2001; **11**(43): 49–54.

7 Ray SA, Srodon PD, Taylor RS *et al.* Reliability of ankle: brachial pressure index measurements by junior doctors. *Br J Surg.* 1994; **81**(2): 188–90.

8 Doubeni CA, Yood RA, Emani S *et al.* Identifying unrecognized peripheral arterial disease among asymptomatic patients in the primary care setting. *Angiology.* 2006; **57**(2): 171–80.

9 Allison MA, Hiatt WR, Hirsch AT *et al.* A high ankle-brachial index is associated with increased cardiovascular disease morbidity and lower quality of life. *J Am Coll Cardiol.* 2008; **51**(13): 1292–8.

10 American Diabetes Association. Peripheral arterial disease in people with diabetes. *Diabetes Care.* 2003; **26**(12): 3333–41.

11 Aboyans V, Ho E, Denenberg JO *et al.* The association between elevated ankle systolic pressures and peripheral occlusive arterial disease in diabetic and nondiabetic subjects. *J Vasc Surg.* 2008; **48**(5): 1197–203.

12 Stein R, Hriljac I, Halperin JL *et al.* Limitation of the resting ankle-brachial index in symptomatic patients with peripheral arterial disease. *Vasc Med.* 2006; **11**(1): 29–33.

13 Kaiser V, Kester AD, Stoffers HE *et al.* The influence of experience on the reproducibility of the ankle-brachial systolic pressure ratio in peripheral arterial occlusive disease. *Eur J Vasc Endovasc Surg.* 1999; **18**(1): 25–9.

14 Goodacre S, Sutton AJ, Sampson FC. Meta-analysis: the value of clinical assessment in the diagnosis of deep venous thrombosis. *Ann Intern Med.* 2005; **143**(2): 129–39.

15 Steg PG, Bhatt DL, Wilson PW *et al.* One year cardiovascular event rates in outpatients with atherothrombosis. *JAMA* 2007; 297: 1197.

16 O'Hare AM, Katz R, Shlipak MG *et al.* Mortality and cardiovascular risk across the ankle-arm index spectrum: results from the Cardiovascular Health Study. *Circulation* 2006; 113: 388.

17 Leng GC, Fowkes FGR, Lee AJ *et al.* Use of ankle brachial pressure index to predict cardiovascular events and death: a cohort study. *BMJ.* 1996; **313**(7070): 1440–3.

11

The management of peripheral arterial disease in primary care

Joanne Whitmore

The scale of the problem

In the United Kingdom, there is a minimum of 720 000 people suffering with symptomatic peripheral arterial disease (PAD)[1] and there are 102 000 newly diagnosed cases of PAD annually.[2] The risk of a cardiovascular event (myocardial infarction [MI], stroke or cardiovascular death) for people with PAD is far greater than the risk of amputation. We know that people with PAD are six times more likely to suffer a stroke or heart attack than those people who do not have PAD.[3] The 1-year risk of dying or being hospitalised as a result of a stroke or heart attack for people with PAD is 21.14%, compared with 15.2% for people with coronary heart disease (CHD).[4]

Indications are that PAD is particularly significant in relation to cardiovascular risk, but despite these statistics PAD is largely unrecognised and, if diagnosed, is frequently poorly managed. The general population are not as aware of the signs of PAD when compared with other aspects of cardiovascular disease (CVD) and commonly put signs and symptoms down to the ageing process. This means that patients present later in the disease process.

> A general practice with a list size of 6000 patients will have approximately 30 symptomatic patients with peripheral arterial disease.

Once patients do present with signs of PAD there is not the same emphasis on diagnosis and management, possibly because PAD is not recognised within the Quality and Outcomes Framework. It is generally agreed that improvements in diagnosis and management would be observed if practices were 'incentivised' to produce PAD registers. In fact, Target PAD (www. targetpad.co.uk) highlights the inclusion of PAD within the Quality and Outcomes Framework as a priority recommendation in their recent report.[5] Their other two recommendations identify emphasis on greater medical and public education and more appropriate prescribing. After looking at the evidence Target PAD also believes at least 23% of cardiovascular events can be prevented by the appropriate management of PAD.

JBS 2[6] guidelines encompass the whole of atherosclerotic CVD, putting equal emphasis on acute coronary syndrome, exertional angina, CVD and peripheral arterial disease. The guidance goes on to say that 'any symptomatic manifestation of atherosclerosis in any vascular territory puts a person at high risk of dying from CVD and thus, would be appropriate to offer the same lifestyle and risk factor management to all people with atherosclerotic disease'. Despite this, the importance of risk factor management is less well appreciated in those with PAD than those with CHD. A number of studies suggest that risk factor management is treated less aggressively for those patients with PAD as opposed to those with CHD.[7]

JBS 2[6] and the National Institute for Health and Clinical Excellence (NICE, or NIHCE)[8] agree that the 10-year risk of a cardiovascular event is high enough for PAD to be treated independently as 'high-risk', thus there is no need to perform a cardiovascular risk assessment on this cohort of patients. They require intensive management of risk factors, pharmacotherapy and should be seen annually in keeping with other 'high-risk' patients on disease registers.

This cohort of patients are a high-risk group and aggressive management of risk factors – smoking, exercise, weight control, cholesterol lowering, blood pressure control, glycaemic control and antiplatelet therapy – will result in real benefits in terms of improved quality of life and a reduction in cardiovascular events. There are simple and effective treatments for prevention of MI and stroke in PAD patients and this chapter will address how to reduce risk in these patients.

Smoking

(*See* Chapter 12, Tackling smoking: role of the GP.)

There are approximately 100 000 deaths that are attributable to smoking each year in the United Kingdom, with smoking accounting for 13% of all cardiovascular deaths.[9] The dominant modifiable risk factor for PAD is smoking and people who do smoke are 10–16 times more likely to develop PAD when compared with people who do not smoke.[10] More than 80% of people with PAD are current or ex-smokers and, interestingly, smokers are 2–3 times more likely to develop lower-extremity PAD than people with coronary artery disease.[11]

Although there are no randomised controlled trials that have assessed the effect of stopping smoking specifically on PAD, observational studies have established that the risks of death, MI and amputation are much greater in those who continue to smoke with a diagnosis of PAD than in those who stop. There is also a relationship between the amount of cigarettes smoked and the severity of PAD.[12]

Studies have shown that patients with intermittent claudication who stop smoking can impact favourably on the severity of rest pain experienced and the severity of claudication. Smoking cessation does not appear to improve walking distance though.

There is a convincing case for the use of pharmacological support to assist patients in smoking cessation. It would be feasible to assume from the observational data that pharmacotherapy alongside a structured smoking cessation programme will reap the best rewards. Further advice and guidance on this can be found in the Public Health NICE Guidance on Smoking Cessation.[13]

Exercise

There is evidence to indicate that a supervised exercise programme is beneficial for people suffering with intermittent claudication. A Cochrane review[14] looked at eight eligible trials. The outcome of this review indicated that a supervised exercise programme produced a significant increase in walking distance – an average improvement of 150 m in most patients at 3-month follow-up.

The reasons for this remain unclear. It is commonly assumed that improvements occur as a result of the growth of new collateral blood vessels but there is inadequate evidence to support this at present.[15] It is more likely to be as a result of improved 'skeletal muscle metabolism, muscle hypertrophy, improvements in endothelial function, or altered gait'.[16]

A joint guideline published by the American College of Cardiology (ACC) and the American Heart Association (AHA)[16] gives the clearest guidance on the type, intensity, duration and frequency required for a beneficial exercise programme. It recommends that a supervised exercise programme should be performed for a minimum of 30–45 minutes, at least three times a week and for a minimum of 12 weeks. The exercise (treadmill walking) must ensure that the patient walks until near-maximal pain is achieved in each session.

TABLE 11.1 Summary of the key elements of a supervised exercise programme

PRIMARY CLINICIAN ROLE
<ul><li>Establish the PAD diagnosis using the ankle-brachial index measurement or other objective vascular laboratory evaluations</li><li>Determine that claudication is the major symptom limiting exercise</li><li>Discuss risk-benefit of claudication therapeutic alternatives including pharmacological, percutaneous, and surgical interventions</li><li>Initiate systemic atherosclerosis risk modification</li><li>Perform treadmill stress testing</li><li>Provide formal referral to a claudication exercise rehabilitation program</li></ul>
EXERCISE GUIDELINES FOR CLAUDICATION*
<ul><li>Warm-up and cool-down period of 5 to 10 minutes each</li></ul>**Types of Exercise**<ul><li>Treadmill and track walking are the most effective exercise for claudication</li><li>Resistance training has conferred benefit to individuals with other forms of cardiovascular disease, and its use, as tolerated, for general fitness is complementary to, but not a substitute for, walking</li></ul>

(*continued*)

EXERCISE GUIDELINES FOR CLAUDICATION* (CONT.)

Intensity

- The initial workload of the treadmill is set to a speed and grade that elicits claudication symptoms within 3 to 5 minutes
- Patients walk at this workload until they achieve claudication of moderate severity, which is then followed by a brief period of standing or sitting rest to permit symptoms to resolve

Duration

- The exercise-rest-exercise pattern should be repeated throughout the exercise session
- The initial duration will usually include 35 minutes of intermittent walking and should be increased by 5 minutes each session until 50 minutes of intermittent walking can be accomplished

Frequency

- Treadmill or track walking 3 to 5 times per week

ROLE OF DIRECT SUPERVISION

- As patients improve their walking ability, the exercise workload should be increased by modifying the treadmill grade or speed (or both) to ensure that there is always the stimulus of claudication pain during the workout
- As patients increase their walking ability, there is the possibility that cardiac signs and symptoms may appear (e.g. dysrhythmia, angina, or ST-segment depression). These events should prompt physician re-evaluation.

Adapted with permission from Stewart KJ, Hiatt WR, Regensteiner JG, Hirsch AT. Medical progress: exercise training for claudication. *N Engl J Med* 2002; 347: 1941–51 © 2002 Massachusetts Medical Society. All rights reserved (62a).

* These general guidelines should be individualized and based on the results of treadmill stress testing and the clinical status of the patient. A full discussion of the exercise precautions for persons with concomitant diseases can be found elsewhere for diabetes (Ruderman N, Devlin JT, Schneider S, Kriska A. *Handbook of Exercise in Diabetes.* Alexandria, VA: American Diabetes Association, 2002) (62b), hypertension (ACSM's Guidelines for Exercise Testing and Prescription. In: Franklin BA, editor. Baltimore, MD: Lippincott, Williams, and Wilkins, 2000) (62c), and coronary artery disease (Guidelines for Cardiac Rehabilitation and Secondary Prevention/American Association of Cardiovascular and Pulmonary Rehabilitation. Champaign, IL: Human Kinetics, 1999) (62d).

Source: ACC/AHA 2005 Practice Guidelines for the management of patients with peripheral arterial disease (lower extremity, renal, mesenteric, and abdominal aortic).[16]

It would not be sufficient to simply advise the patient to exercise more; benefits have only been observed within a formal, structured exercise programme. Unfortunately, there is a distinct lack of structured exercise programmes for PAD sufferers in the United Kingdom. Utilising and adapting existing cardiac rehabilitation and acute coronary syndrome exercise programmes is a potential solution, as these programmes have the expertise and resource needed to support a structured exercise programme.

Weight reduction and cardioprotective diet

There are no studies investigating weight reduction in patients with PAD although obesity (classed as a body mass index $> 30\,kg/m^2$) is associated with higher levels of cholesterol, blood pressure and blood glucose. Obesity is also associated with an increased risk of CVD and death caused by CVD. People who are overweight or obese should be offered appropriate advice and support in line with NICE clinical guidance on obesity.[17]

Advice can be given on a cardio protective diet. The main elements of a cardioprotective diet are:

- total fat intake should be 30% or less of the total energy intake
- saturated fat intake should be 10% or less of total energy intake
- dietary cholesterol should be less than 300 mg per day
- where possible, saturated fat should be replaced with monounsaturated and polyunsaturated fats
- eat at least five portions of fruit and vegetables each day
- eat at least two portions of fish per week including a portion of oily fish.

Further advice can be found at the Eat Well website (http://eatwell.gov.uk/healthydiet).

Pharmacotherapy

The Scottish Intercollegiate Guidelines Network (SIGN)[7] suggest that the control of risk factors alone is inadequate in reducing risk back to normal in patients with PAD and advise a combination of lifestyle modification and pharmacotherapy. Epidemiological studies have shown that even after taking into consideration cardiovascular risk factors patients with PAD are still at an increased risk from having a cardiovascular event.

Lipid-lowering therapy

Treatment with a statin should be offered to *all* patients diagnosed with PAD *unless contraindicated*.

A recent Cochrane review[18] considering the effects of lipid-lowering therapy on all-cause mortality, cardiovascular events and local disease progression in patients with lower limb PAD concluded that lipid-lowering therapy is effective in reducing cardiovascular mortality and morbidity and advocates the use of a statin in people with PAD with a total cholesterol of at least 3.5 mmol/Litre. The evidence was not as clear in people with a total cholesterol of less than 3.5 mmol/Litre.

The review included 18 randomised controlled trials involving over 10 000 people, three-quarters of whom were men. Statins were the only drug that had consistent clear evidence of the beneficial effect on total cardiovascular events, total coronary events and stroke.

The majority of the evidence points towards simvastatin as the statin of choice; however, this may be because simvastatin was the drug used in the majority of studies. A PAD subgroup of the Heart Protection Study[19] showed that simvastatin 40 mg significantly lowered cardiovascular event rates by 22%. A retrospective study of the 4S Trial[20] revealed that simvastatin reduced the risk of both new and worsening claudication, while two other studies[21,22] found that both simvastatin and atorvastatin significantly increase pain-free walking time. There is some data to suggest that the non-cholesterol-lowering properties of statins are responsible for improving leg function in patients with PAD.[23,24]

Despite the evidence, a recent review[25] highlighted that only 47% of patients referred for amputation had been prescribed a statin and the AGATHA study[26] found that only two-thirds of dyslipidaemic patients with or at risk of vascular disease were receiving lipid-lowering therapy.

There are no cholesterol treatment targets relating specifically to PAD, but the lipid modification guidelines produced by NICE[8] advocate that simvastatin (40 mg) should be used in the first instance for the secondary prevention of CVD. If a target total cholesterol of 4 mmol/Litre and low-density lipoprotein of 2 mmol/Litre is not reached, a higher dose of simvastatin or a drug of similar efficacy and acquisition should be considered. NICE do acknowledge, however, that more than half of patients will not achieve these targets.

With the launch of generic simvastatin, there is a greater opportunity to prescribe cost-effective statin. The pace of switch from other statins to simvastatin is set to accelerate because of its inclusion as percentage of prescribing – an incentive indicator by primary care trusts. Some primary care trusts have given a resource pack as a guidance to general practitioners about the switch-over, e.g. atorvastatin 10 mg to simvastation 40 mg. Some have provided services of a pharmacist free of charge to help the 'pressed-for-time' general practitioners. There is a growing pressure on English primary care trusts to achieve 69% on low-cost statin prescribing (at the time of writing this book).

What to do if cholesterol targets not reached with statin prescribing:

- check the compliance of the drug by looking into the prescribing screen – when was the last script issued?
- titrate the dose by doubling the strength, adding a cholesterol absorption inhibitor (ezetimibe) or switching to a more potent statin (atorvastatin)
- start fibrate
- make sure patient is adhering to lifestyle measures
- consider a trial of highly concentrated, licensed omega-3 fish oils (as per NICE guidelines)
- refer to lipid specialist.

Antiplatelet therapy

The Antithrombotic Trialists' (ATT) Collaboration conducted a meta-analysis[27] where they analysed 195 trials comparing a variety of antiplatelets against a control group in patients who were at increased risk of occlusive arterial disease. The analysis observed that antiplatelet therapy reduced the risk of MI, stroke or cardiovascular death by one-quarter.

The PAD subgroup analysis of 42 trials (9214 patients) showed similar reductions (23%). These benefits were seen across the PAD spectrum, from patients who suffered with intermittent claudication as well as those patients undergoing peripheral angioplasty or bypass surgery.

The ATT[27] observed that aspirin did not improve claudication but it did delay the rate of progression. The benefit of aspirin in reducing the frequency of thrombotic events in the peripheral arteries and overall cardiovascular mortality was also shown.

There was also some debate over the dosage of aspirin to be given but studies seem to show that 75–150 mg given long term is at least as effective as higher daily doses (which could potentially increase the risk of adverse events).

It should be recognised, however, that the analysis evaluated multiple antiplatelet agents and questions have been raised as to whether the overall benefit of antiplatelet agents, particularly aspirin, in PAD may have 'been driven by therapeutic regimens rather than Aspirin'.[28]

Further doubts have been raised following the publication of the POPADAD trial (2008),[29] which looked at the administration of aspirin in patients with PAD and diabetes. The study concluded that there was no benefit for aspirin therapy. Interestingly, Berger et al.[28] also highlighted the fact that the US Food and Drug Administration have not licensed aspirin to treat PAD due to insufficient evidence and the recent Transatlantic Inter-Society Consensus (TASC II)[1] guideline only issued a level-C recommendation for the administration of aspirin in patients with isolated PAD.

Aspirin is still the most widely studied antiplatelet but there have not been enough trials specifically looking at aspirin in PAD patients to conclusively say that aspirin is of benefit in preventing heart attack, stroke or cardiovascular death. Berger et al.'s[28] meta-analysis assessed the effect of aspirin on the risks of cardiovascular events. It looked at 18 trials including 5269 patients with PAD. The analysis concluded that there was a statistically non-significant decrease in cardiovascular events and a statistically significant reduction in the secondary endpoint of non-fatal stroke. It is acknowledged, though, that the study lacked statistical power and suggests that further randomised controlled trials are needed.

The lack of statistical power in Berger et al.'s meta-analysis supports the fact that there is a lack of clinical trial data available to inform the management of PAD. McDermott et al.'s[30] comments on the study advise that this analysis should not change current clinical practice or guidelines relating to the administration of aspirin in patients with PAD and agree that more high-quality trials are needed. The results of the ongoing aspirin in the asymptomatic atherosclerosis clinical trial[31] are eagerly awaited.

Clopidogrel

Clopidogrel was found to be slightly more effective than aspirin in the CHARISMA study.[32] Furthermore, the CAPRIE study[33] discovered that the greatest benefit was observed in the PAD subgroup analysis of 6452 patients. It showed a 23.8% Relative Risk Reduction (RRR) in MI, stroke or cardiovascular death in favour of clopidogrel (75 mg) versus aspirin (325 mg).

SIGN[7] guidelines on PAD acknowledge that the cost-effectiveness of clopidogrel in patients with PAD has not been suitably demonstrated in relation to preventing cardiovascular death. The expense of clopidogrel in comparison with aspirin means that it is not the first-choice therapy in the United Kingdom.

There is no evidence to support dual antiplatelet therapy.

Anticoagulants

Anticoagulants are not indicated in the medical management of PAD unless there is a specific condition, such as atrial fibrillation, that would warrant their use. There is a suggestion that anticoagulants may have a role to play after bypass surgery.

There is no indication for warfarin in the non-critical phase of PAD. The risks of bleeding outweigh the potential benefits.

Other

There does not appear to be any benefit in using dipyridamole. It remains controversial and is not recommended in any of the major guidelines.

Picotamide, which inhibits thromboxane A2 synthase and blocks thromboxane A2 receptors, was shown to significantly reduce mortality in patients with PAD and diabetes.[34] Several less-well-known antiplatelet drugs, such as triflusal and ketanserin, have not been shown to be superior to aspirin for preventing systemic complications in patients with PAD.

Antihypertensive therapy

There have been some concerns about prescribing antihypertensive medications in the presence of PAD. It has been thought that these drugs, especially beta blockers, could induce further vasoconstriction in the peripheries, leading to worsening ischaemia.

The Cochrane review[35] concluded that, in patients with PAD, there was insufficient evidence to suggest that beta blockers should not be prescribed. However, it also acknowledged that there was a lack of robust studies that demonstrate a definitive outcome. Beta blockers would not be first-line treatment in the United Kingdom anyway, if we were to follow the British Hypertension Society's guidelines[36] and if beta blockers were to be considered, the newer agents would deem this issue as irrelevant now.[7]

The Cochrane update[18] on the original 2003 guidance on the treatment of hypertension in PAD looked at a further four randomised controlled trials. The review concluded that the evidence for the use of antihypertensive medication in patients with PAD is still lacking and it was unable to say whether there are significant benefits or risks involved. It does reinforce the overwhelming evidence for treating hypertension per se though.

There is some evidence that ACE (angiotensin-converting enzyme) inhibitors are of particular benefit in patients with PAD. The HOPE study[37] enrolled 4051 patients with PAD, of which 1966 were assigned ramipril. A Relative Risk Reduction (RRR) of 25% was observed in cardiovascular events in this arm of the study.

Both SIGN guidance[7] and ACC/AHA guidance[16] advocate the treatment of hypertension in patients with PAD, stating that most people would be able to tolerate therapy without a worsening of symptoms. All antihypertensive therapies are effective in reducing cardiovascular events and there are clear guidelines in the United Kingdom around the management of blood pressure. In light of the lack of evidence relating specifically to PAD, direction should be sought from the British Hypertension Society's guidelines.[36]

Homocysteine

Patients with PAD have been found to have an increased level of homocysteine and this has been implicated as an independent risk factor for developing atherosclerotic disease.

There have been a small number of observational studies assessing the effect of both folate and vitamin B_6 supplementation on patients with PAD. A recent meta-analysis[38] concluded that, although PAD sufferers have significantly higher levels of homocysteine, there was insufficient evidence for folate supplementation in this cohort of patients.

> **KEY POINTS**
> - Incidence of PAD increases with age.
> - Smoking is the single biggest risk factor.
> - Only one-third of all patients with PAD present with classical symptoms of intermittent claudication.

Further reading

- The Vascular Society of Great Britain and Ireland. *The Provision of Services for Patients with Vascular Disease* 2009. Available at: www.vascularsociety.org.uk/ library/vascular-society-publications/doc_download/65-revised-provision-of-vascular-services-2004.html (accessed 10 March 2011).
- Primary care service framework peripheral arterial disease: Available at www.pcc.nhs.uk/uploads/primary_care_service_frameworks/2009/pcsf_pad_finalv2_doc.pdf (accessed 10 March 2011).

References

1 Norgren L, Hiatt WR, Dormandy JA *et al*. Inter-Society Consensus for the management of Peripheral Arterial Disease (TASC II). *Eur J Vasc Endovasc Surg.* 2007; **33**(Suppl. 1): S1–75.

2 National Institute for Health and Clinical Excellence. *Clopidogrel and Dipyridamole for the prevention of atherosclerotic events: NICE technical appraisal 90*. London: NIHCE; 2005. Available at www.nice.org.uk/TA/90 (accessed July 2010).

3 Tierney S, Fennessy F, Bouchier-Hayes D. ABC of arterial and vascular disease. Secondary prevention of peripheral vascular disease. *BMJ.* 2000; **320**: 1262–5.

4 Steg PG, Bhatt DL, Wilson PW *et al*. One-year cardiovascular event rates in outpatients with atherothrombosis. *JAMA.* 2007; **297**(11): 1197–206.

5 Stansby G, Belch J. Dragging their feet: the cost of suboptimal treatment for patients diagnosed with peripheral arterial disease. *Prim Care Cardiovasc J.* 2008; 1(Suppl. 2): S4–11.

6 British Cardiac Society, British Hypertension Society, Diabetes UK *et al*. JBS 2: Joint British Societies' guidelines on prevention of cardiovascular disease in clinical practice. *Heart.* 2005; 91(Suppl. 5): v1–52.

7 Scottish Intercollegiate Guidelines Network (SIGN). *Diagnosis and Management of Peripheral Arterial Disease: a national clinical guideline*. Publication No 89, 2006. Edinburgh: SIGN.

8 National Institute for Health and Clinical Excellence. *Lipid Modification: cardiovascular risk assessment and the modification of blood lipids for the primary and secondary prevention of cardiovascular disease; NICE guideline 67*. London: NIHCE; 2008. www.nice.org.uk/CG67 (accessed July 2010).

9 Action on Smoking and Health. *Beyond Smoking Kills*. London: Action on Smoking and Health; 2008.

10 Scott M, Stansby G. 10 steps before you refer for peripheral arterial disease. *BJC*. 2009; **16**(6): 288–91.

11 Price JF, Mowbray PI, Lee AJ *et al*. Relationship between smoking and cardiovascular risk factors in the development of peripheral arterial disease and coronary artery disease: Edinburgh Artery Study. *Eur Heart J*; 1999, **20**(5): 344–53.

12 Hankey GJ, Norman PE, Eikelboom JW. Medical treatment of peripheral arterial disease. *JAMA*. 2006; **295**(5); 547–53.

13 National Institute for Health and Clinical Excellence. *Smoking Cessation Services: NICE guidance 10*. London: NIHCE; 2008. www.nice.org.uk/PH10 (accessed July 2010).

14 Bendermacher BL, Willigendael EM, Teijink JA *et al*. Supervised exercise therapy versus non-supervised exercise therapy for intermittent claudication. *Cochrane Database Syst Rev*. 2006; **2**. CD005263.

15 Stewart KJ, Hiatt WR, Regensteiner JG *et al*. Exercise training for claudication. *N Engl J Med*. 2002; **347**(24): 1941–51.

16 Hirsch AT, Haskal ZJ, Hertzer NR *et al*. ACC/AHA 2005 Practice Guidelines for the management of patients with peripheral arterial disease (lower extremity, renal, mesenteric, and abdominal aortic): a collaborative report from the American Association for Vascular Surgery/Society for Vascular Surgery, Society for Cardiovascular Angiography and Interventions, Society for Vascular Medicine and Biology, Society of Interventional Radiology, and the ACC/AHA Task Force on Practice Guidelines (Writing Committee to Develop Guidelines for the Management of Patients With Peripheral Arterial Disease): endorsed by the American Association of Cardiovascular and Pulmonary Rehabilitation; National Heart, Lung, and Blood Institute; Society for Vascular Nursing; TransAtlantic Inter-Society Consensus; and Vascular Disease Foundation. *Circulation* 2006; **113**(11): e463–654.

17 National Institute for Health and Clinical Excellence. *Guidance on the prevention, identification, assessment and management of overweight and obesity in adults and children. NICE guidance 43.* London: NIHCE; 2006. www.nice.org.uk/CG43 (accessed July 2010).

18 Lane DA, Lip GY. Treatment of hypertension in peripheral arterial disease. *Cochrane Database Syst Rev.* 2009; **4**. CD003075.

19 Heart Protection Study Collaborative Group. MRC/BHF Heart Protection Study of cholesterol lowering with simvastatin in 20,536 high-risk individuals: a randomised placebo-controlled trial. *Lancet.* 2002; **360**(9326): 7–22.

20 Pedersen TR, Kjekshus J, Pyörälä K *et al.* Effect of simvastatin on ischaemic signs and symptoms in the Scandinavian simvastatin survival study (4S). *Am J Cardiol.* 1998; **81**(3): 333–5.

21 Aronow WS, Nayak D, Woodworth S *et al.* Effect of simvastatin versus placebo on exercise treadmill time until the onset of intermittent claudication in older patients with peripheral arterial disease at six months and at one year after treatment. *Am J Cardiol.* 2003; **92**(6): 711–12.

22 Mohler ER, Hiatt WR, Creager MA. Cholesterol reduction with atorvastatin improves walking distance in patients with peripheral arterial disease. *Circulation.* 2003; **108**(12): 1481–6.

23 McDermott MM, Guralnik JM, Greenland P *et al.* Statin use and leg functioning in patients with and without lower-extremity peripheral arterial disease. *Circulation.* 2003; **107**(5): 757–61.

24 Mondillo S, Ballo P, Barbati R *et al.* Effects of simvastatin on walking performance and symptoms of intermittent claudication in hypercholesterolemic patients with peripheral arterial disease. *Am J Med.* 2003; **114**(5): 359–64.

25 Bradley L, Kirker SG. Secondary prevention of arteriosclerosis in lower limb vascular amputees: a missed opportunity. *Eur J Vasc Endovasc Surg.* 2006; **32**(5): 491–3.

26 Fowkes FG, Low LP, Tuta S *et al.* Ankle-brachial index and extent of atherothrombosis in 8891 patients with or at risk of vascular disease: results of the international AGATHA study. *Eur Heart J.* 2006; **27**(15): 1861–7.

27 Antithrombotic Trialists' Collaboration. Collaborative metaanalysis of randomised trials of antiplatelet therapy for prevention of death, myocardial infarction, and stroke in high risk patients. *BMJ.* 2002; **324**(7329): 71–86.

28 Berger JS, Krantz MJ, Kittelson JM *et al.* Aspirin for the prevention of cardiovascular events in patients with peripheral artery disease: a meta-analysis of randomized trials. *JAMA.* 2009; **301**(18): 1909–19.

29 Belch J, MacCuish A, Campbell I, *et al.* The prevention of progression of arterial disease and diabetes (POPADAD) trial: factorial randomised placebo controlled trial of aspirin and antioxidants in patients with diabetes and asymptomatic peripheral arterial disease. *BMJ.* 2008; 337: a1840. DOI: 10.1136/bmj.a1840.

30 McDermott MM, Criqui MH. Aspirin and secondary prevention in peripheral artery disease: a perspective for the early 21st century. *JAMA.* 2009; **301**(18): 1927–8.

31 Price JF, Stewart MC, Deary IJ *et al.* Low dose aspirin and cognitive function in middle aged to elderly adults: randomised controlled trial. *BMJ.* 2008; 337: a1198. DOI: 10.1136/bmj.a1198.

32 Bhatt D L, Topol E J, Clopidogrel for High Atherothrombotic Risk and Ischaemic Stabilization, Management, and Avoidance Executive Committee. Clopidogrel added to aspirin versus aspirin alone in secondary prevention and high-risk primary prevention: rationale and design of the Clopidogrel for High Atherothrombotic Risk and Ischaemic Stabilization, Management, and Avoidance (CHARISMA) trial. *Am Heart J.* 2004, **148**(2): 263–8.

33 No authors listed. A randomized, blinded trial of clopidogrel versus aspirin in patients at risk of ischaemic events (CAPRIE): CAPRIE Steering Committee. *Lancet.* 1996; **348**(9038): 1329–39.

34 Neri Serneri GG, Coccheri S, Marubini E *et al.* Picotamide, a combined inhibitor of thromboxane A2 synthase and receptor, reduces 2-year mortality in diabetics with peripheral arterial disease: the DAVID study. *Eur Heart J.* 2004; **25**(20): 1845–52.

35 Lip GY, Makin AJ. Treatment of hypertension in peripheral arterial disease. *Cochrane Database Syst Rev.* 2003; **3**: CD003075.

36 Williams B, Poulter NR, Brown MJ *et al.* Guidelines for management of hypertension: report of the fourth working party of the British Hypertension Society, 2004-BHS IV. *J Hum Hypertens.* 2004; **18**(3): 139–85.

37 Yusuf S, Sleight P, Pogue J *et al.* Effects of an angiotensin-converting-enzyme inhibitor, ramipril, on cardiovascular events in high-risk patients. The Heart Outcomes Prevention Evaluation Study Investigators. *N Engl J Med.* 2000; **342**(3): 145–53.

38 Khandanpour N, Loke YK, Meyer FJ *et al.* Homocysteine and peripheral arterial disease: systematic review and meta-analysis. *Eur J Vasc Endovasc Surg.* 2009; **38**(3): 316–22.

12

Tackling smoking: role of the GP

Smoking cessation guidelines recommend that all healthcare professionals should check the smoking status of their patients at least once a year and advise smoking cessation. The electronic patient record system automatically requests this information. Since the introduction of the Quality and Outcomes Framework, with incentives to record smoking status and advice given, all general practitioners (GPs) provide advice opportunistically during routine consultations or as part of chronic disease management.

In total there are 60 quality points relating to recording of smoking and advising stopping smoking.

Smoking indicators

TABLE 12.1 Quality and Outcomes Framework Guidance for GMS Contract 2009/10

INDICATOR	POINT	PAYMENT STAGES
Ongoing management		
Smoking 3: The percentage of patients with any or any combination of the following conditions: coronary heart disease, stroke or TIA, hypertension, diabetes, COPD, CKD, asthma, schizophrenia, bipolar effective disorder or any other psychoses whose notes record smoking status in the previous 15 months	30	40%–90%

(*continued*)

INDICATOR	POINT	PAYMENT STAGES
Smoking 4: The percentage of patients with any or any combination of the following conditions: coronary heart disease, stroke or TIA, hypertension, diabetes, COPD, CKD, asthma, schizophrenia, bipolar effective disorder or any other psychoses who smoke whose notes contain a record that smoking cessation advice or referral to a specialist service, where available, has been offered within the previous 15 months	30	40%–90%

Source: Quality and Outcomes Framework Guidance for GMS Contract 2009/10.

Preferred Read codes

- 137I – never smoked.
- 137L – ex-smoker.
- 137R – smoker.
- 8CAL – smoking cessation advice.

The code 'never smoked' needs to be entered only once. If the code 'non-smoker' (not smoked for 12 months) has been used it will need to be removed or repeated each year as it is considered similar to the code 'ex-smoker'.

Role of the general practitioner

A stop smoking intervention should always be offered routinely, regardless of whether a smoker shows an interest in stopping smoking.[1]

Currently 73% of smokers want to stop smoking, and 79% of smokers have tried and failed.[2]

The data from the General Household Survey 2007 shows that 21% of adults are smoking. However, the rate in manual groups is high – 29% in Great Britain.[3] The Public Service Agreement (PSA) target for smoking is to reduce the adult smoking rate to 21% or less, and 26% or less in routine and manual groups by 2010.[4]

GPs are ideally placed to provide brief smoking cessation advice.[5]

Brief smoking cessation advice[5]

The Five As

- *Ask:* ask and record smoking status, e.g. smoker, non-smoker or an ex-smoker.
- *Advise:* all smokers should be advised of the risks involved with smoking and the value of stopping. This should be recorded by computer and/or in written records.
- *Assess:* all smokers should be assessed regarding their willingness to stop by asking, 'Have you ever tried to stop?' and 'Do you want to stop?'
- *Assist:* provide information through self-help leaflets; help them decide on a stop date, advise on smoking cessation medication, issue a prescription and refer to local smoking cessation service, if available in your area.
- *Arrange follow-up:* if a patient is not interested in stopping smoking give a follow-up appointment to discuss smoking again. Let them know that support is available if they change their mind.

Most primary care trusts providing a smoking cessation service will have their own form to record the service provision to the patient.

Treatment

Behavioural therapy

This can be provided with or without the pharmacological interventions. The greater the frequency of the support, the greater the success.[6]

Alternative treatment

Alternative treatment includes hypnosis, acupuncture, acupressure, laser therapy, electrostimulation and anxiolytics. These are not available through the National Health Service because of the lack of evidence on effectiveness.

Pharmacotherapy

Nicotine replacement therapy (NRT)

This is an extremely safe and well-tolerated treatment. This can be prescribed in the form of skin patches, chewing gum, lozenges, nasal spray or inhalator and is normally used for a period of 6–12 weeks. NRT can be

OLDHAM STOP SMOKING SERVICE

NHS
Oldham Community
Health Services

MONITORING & EVALUATION FORM		
ADVISER DETAILS:		
Department/Ward:	Location/setting:	
Name:	Venue:	
Contact Tel. No.:	Adviser code/ref:	

CLIENT DETAILS:		
Surname:	First Name:	Mr/Mrs/Ms/Other
Address:		
Postcode:	NHS ID No.:	
Daytime Tel. No.:	Mobile No.:	
Alternative contact number (friend/relative):		
Date of Birth:	Age (in years):	Gender: Male/Female
Exempt from prescription charge Y / N	Pregnant Y / N	Breast feeding Y / N

Occupation code   Full-time student ☐   Never worked/long term unemployed ☐   Retired ☐
(see reverse for   Home carer ☐   Sick/disabled and unable to work ☐   Managerial/professional ☐
further information)   Intermediate ☐   Routine & manual ☐   Unable to code ☐

ETHNIC GROUP: *(please tick relevant group)*

a) White	☐	b) Mixed	☐	c) Asian or Asian British	☐
British	☐	White and Black Caribbean	☐	Indian	☐
Irish	☐	White and Black African	☐	Pakistani	☐
Other white background	☐	White and Asian	☐	Bangladeshi	☐
		Other mixed groups	☐	Other Asian background	☐
d) Black or Black British	☐	e) Other ethnic groups	☐	f) Other not stated	☐
Caribbean	☐	Chinese	☐		
African	☐	Other ethnic group	☐		
Other black background	☐				

HOW CLIENT HEARD ABOUT THE SERVICE: *(please tick relevant box)*

GP	☐	Friend/relative	☐	Pharmacy	☐
Other health professional	☐	Advertising	☐	Other *(please specify)*	☐
Been on before	☐				

Agreed quit date:	Date of last tobacco use:	Date of 4 wk follow-up:

TYPE OF INTERVENTION DELIVERED: *(please tick all relevant boxes)*

Closed group	☐	Telephone support	☐	Other *(please specify)*	☐
Open (rolling) group	☐	Couple/family	☐		
One to one support	☐	Drop-in-clinic	☐		

TYPE OF PHARMACOLOGICAL SUPPORT USED: *(please tick all relevant boxes. Use 1 or 2 to indicate consecutive use of more than one medication – e.g. Champix followed by NRT product)*

None	☐	Zyban	☐	NRT – Gum	☐
NRT – Lozenge	☐	NRT – Inhaler	☐	NRT – Patch	☐
NRT – Microtab	☐	NRT – Spray	☐	Champix	☐

TREATMENT OUTCOME:

Quit CO verified ☐	Quit self report ☐	Not Quit ☐	Lost to follow up ☐

Adviser signature	Client signature *(indicating consent to treatment and follow-up and pass on of outcome data to GP and DoH)*

*This information is stored for a maximum of 18 months. It is confidential, not passed on to other bodies and is used only to provide statistical data.

FIGURE 12.1 Oldham's Stop Smoking Service

prescribed for up to 9 months if needed. These forms are all equally effective and choice can be patient-led.[7]

NRT works by delivering a controlled dose of nicotine in the body with none of the harmful agents that are in tobacco smoke.[8]

The various preparations are: Nicopatch 7 mg, 14 mg, 21 mg; Nicorette patch 5 mg, 10 mg, 15 mg; Nicotinell TTS 10 (7 mg/24 hrs), Nicotinell TTS 20 (14 mg/24 hrs), Nicotinell TTS 30 (21 mg/24 hrs); Niquitin patches 21 mg. A high-strength Nicorette 25 mg patch delivers 25 mg of nicotine over 16 hours and has been shown to reduce withdrawal symptoms.

The most common side effects are gastrointestinal disturbance, head-aches, dizziness and dry mouth, and, less frequently, palpitations and skin irritation with patches, irritation of nose and throat with nasal spray and mouth ulceration with gums and lozenges.

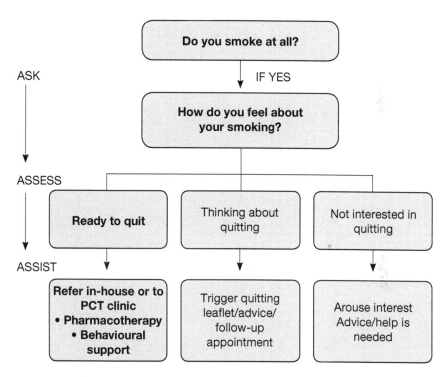

FIGURE 12.2 Opportunistic assessment of a smoker's readiness to quit: Help 2 Quit approach

SCAPE (Smoking Cessation Action in Primary CarE)

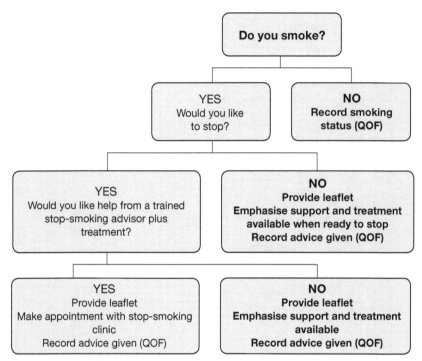

This algorithm has been adopted from the Smoking Cessation Action in Primary Care (SCAPE) Taskforce.

FIGURE 12.3 A simple smoking cessation intervention in primary care

Two models used in primary care are:

- *Help 2 Quit Model:* this model was developed in Shropshire and was established in 1995.
- *H2Q:* this is a nurse-led programme and can be easily delivered in a primary care setting.

Bupropion

This is a prescription drug, taken once daily for 6 days and then twice daily for 7–9 weeks.[9] This is a non-nicotine tablet that works by breaking the addiction cycle. Bupropion was first licensed as an atypical antidepressant and then was discovered to be effective in smoking cessation therapy.[10]

Highly motivated patients who stop smoking during the standard 7-week bupropion programme are likely to maintain abstinence as long as they continue to take the drug, at least for 1 year. In this multicentre randomised double-blind placebo-controlled trial, 55.1% of the patients treated with bupropion were not smoking at the end of 1 year as compared to 42.3% in the placebo group.[11]

The most common side effects are dry mouth, insomnia and nauseous feeling. It is contraindicated in pregnancy, breastfeeding, history of epilepsy, seizures and eating disorders.

For full product information refer to Zyban (bupropion).[9]

The National Institute for Health and Clinical Excellence (NICE, or NIHCE) has published guidance on the use of NRT and bupropion, recommending either for smokers who wish to stop smoking.[12]

Varenicline (Champix/Pfizer)

Varenicline is an effective treatment for smoking cessation. It is a partial nicotine receptor agonist that targets alpha-4 beta-2 nicotinic acetylcholine receptor subtypes and is licensed as an aid to stopping smoking.[13] It is available in 0.5 mg and 1 mg tablets.

- Days 1–3: 0.5 mg once daily.
- Days 4–7: 0.5 mg twice daily.
- Day 8 till end: 1 mg twice daily.

It is a 12-week course but can be given for a further 12 weeks to those who feel they need it.[13]

Dosing should start 1 week before the planned cessation date and tablets should be taken after eating and with a full glass of water.[13]

It is not recommended for children or adolescents less than 18 years of age.[13] It can increase the chances of long-term abstinence by twofold to threefold versus placebo.[14]

It is generally well tolerated but should be used with caution in people with decreased renal function, epilepsy, schizophrenia and bipolar disorders.[15] There have been reports of depression and suicidal tendencies in patients taking varenicline. The drug should be stopped immediately if the patient shows signs and symptoms of depression or agitation.[16]

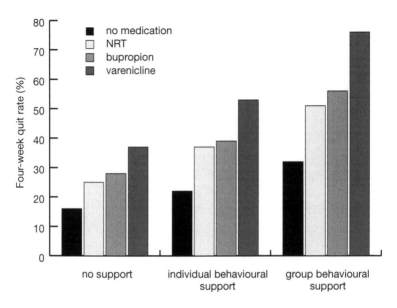

FIGURE 12.4 Effectiveness of pharmacotherapy and support options. The relative impact of a variety of evidence-based stop smoking interventions and pharmacotherapies upon 4-week quit period.[17]

The future

A new National Health Service centre for smoking cessation and training to provide evidence-based service has been set up in 2009–10. It will provide key services, gold standard training programmes and evidence-based best practice delivery models.

Electronic cigarettes (e-cigarette)

One of the most recent products in the market, these are battery operated devices and are meant to reduce the concentrations of toxic compounds in smoke, helping smokers to give up.

To date, the research and clinical trials in humans are lacking. Food and Drug Administration's (FDA) analysis showed that with each puff cartridges emitted different amounts of nicotine, propylene glycol (a generally safe antifreeze found in various cosmetics and foods), diethylene glycol (toxic liquid involved in mass poisoning) and powerful carcinogen N-nitrosamine (chemically related to nicotine and other tobacco alkaloids). Tobacco-specific impurities anabasine, myosmine and B-nicotyrine were also detected by the

FDA but HNZ (Health New Zealand) and Demokriots (a publically funded Greek research institute) did not report these chemicals.[18]

Useful websites

For patients – helplines

- www.gosmokefree.co.uk (England)
- www.canstopsmoking.com (Scotland)
- www.stopsmokingwales.com (Wales)
- www.spacetobreathe.org.uk (Ireland)

For GPs

- Action on Smoking and Health (ASH) provides publications and fact sheets (www.ash.org.uk).
- The British Heart Foundation produces leaflets and literature to help smokers (www.bhf.org.uk).
- GASP Smokefree Services produces leaflets, books and posters (www.gasp.org.uk).
- Smoking Cessation Services (www.scsm.org).

Summary

NICE recommends that all smokers should be encouraged to quit. Most smokers claim that they want to quit (67%)[19] but those who are not sure or cannot decide should be advised to consider quitting and to seek help in the future. NICE recommends that patients are offered a referral to a smoking cessation clinic but if the patient is not willing or is unable to attend, the GP or practice nurse should offer pharmacotherapy and provide support.[20]

KEY POINTS

- Quality and Outcomes Framework points are available for recording smoking status and offering advice.
- It is a team effort – all primary healthcare professionals, as and when the opportunity arises, should give advice on stopping smoking.
- Treatment should be offered within the practice or by a referral to a smoking cessation clinic.

References

1 Anczak JD, Nogler RA. Tobacco cessation in primary care: maximizing intervention strategies. *Clin Med Res.* 2003; **1**(3): 201–16.

2 Lader D. *Smoking-Related Behaviour and Attitudes, 2007.* Cardiff: Office for National Statistics; 2008.

3 Robinson S, Lader D. *Smoking and Drinking among Adults, 2007.* Newport: Office for National Statistics; 2008.

4 HM Treasury. *2004 Spending Review.* London: HM Treasury; 2004.

5 West R, McNeill A, Raw M. Smoking cessation guidelines for health professionals: an update. Health Education Authority. *Thorax.* 2000; **55**(12): 987–99.

6 Kottke TE, Battista RN, DeFriese GH *et al.* Attributes of successful smoking cessation interventions in medical practice: a meta-analysis of 39 controlled trials. *JAMA.* 1988; **259**(19): 2883–9.

7 Stead LF, Perera R, Bullen C *et al.* Nicotine replacement therapy for smoking cessation. *Cochrane Database Syst Rev.* 2008; January 23; (**1**): CD000146.

8 Committee on Safety of Medicines, Medicines and Healthcare products Regulatory Agency (MHRA). *Report of the Committee on Safety of Medicines Working Group on Nicotine Replacement Therapy.* London: MHRA; 2005.

9 Bupropion MedlinePlus DrugInformation. www.nlm.nih.gov/medlineplus/druginfo/meds/a695033.html (accessed 10 March 2011).

10 Roddy E. Bupropion and other non-nicotine pharmacotherapies. *BMJ.* 2004; **328**(7438): 509–11.

11 Thomas A, Barringer, Elizabeth M *et al.* Does long term bupropion use prevent smoking relapse after initial success at quitting smoking. *Journal of Family Practice.* February 2002.

12 National Institute for Health and Clinical Excellence. *Smoking Cessation: bupropion and nicotine replacement therapy (replaced by PH10): NICE technology appraisal 39.* www.nice.org.uk/TA39. London: NICE; 2002 (accessed 18 March 2011).

13 Pfizer Limited. *Varenicline.* www.pfizer.com/files/products/ppi_chantix.pdf (accessed 10 March 2011).

14 Nides M, Glover ED, Reus VI *et al.* Varenicline versus bupropion SR or placebo for smoking cessation: a pooled analysis. *Am J Health Behav.* 2008; **32**(6): 664–75.

15 Champix (Varenicline) 25 November 2008. www.netdoctor.co.uk/medicines/100005109.html (accessed 10 March 2011).

16 Champix Information and Stopping Smoking 14 January 2007 www.champix
info.co.uk (accessed 10 March 2011).

17 Department of Health. *NHS Stop Smoking Services: service and monitoring guidance 2010/11*. March 2009. Available at: www.dh.gov.uk/en/Publications andstatistics/Publications/PublicationsPolicyAndGuidance/DH_109696 (accessed 10 March 2011).

18 Flouris AD, Oikonomou DN. Electronic cigarettes: miracle or menace? *BMJ*. 2010; 340: c311.

19 The NHS Information Centre, Lifestyles Statistics. August 2010. *Statistics on NHS Stop Smoking Services: England, April 2009–March 2010*. Available at: www.ic.nhs.uk/webfiles/publications/Health%20and%20Lifestyles/SSS_ 2009_10_revised.pdf (accessed 25 March 2011).

20 National Institute for Health and Clinical Excellence. *Brief Intervention and Referral for Smoking Cessation in Primary Care and Other Settings*. Quick reference guide. March 2006.

13

PAD: primary care service framework

NHS Primary Care Commissioning, the Department of Health's policy implementation body, has circulated a primary care service framework for peripheral arterial disease to all primary care trusts.[1]

The NHS Health Check programme consists of a series of clinical and cost-effective tests for identifying people with diabetes, heart disease, a stroke and kidney disease. Peripheral arterial disease (PAD) is not a part of this programme. The new service framework feels that PAD should be a part of this programme because it has the same aetiology as coronary artery disease or a stroke and has a significant impact on health.

The main purpose of the service framework is to deliver a high-quality service in primary care for symptomatic patients with PAD. This includes early diagnosis, management of symptoms and risk reduction.[1] The framework raises the profile of PAD and is deliverable if commissioners, providers and practitioners work together with the necessary background knowledge. Patient and public involvement will be crucial in service provision.

PAD framework[1]

- Establishing a disease register, identifying early PAD and intervene to prevent disease progression and complications related directly to PAD.
- Targeting symptomatic middle-aged 50 to 69-year-old male and female

patients with history of smoking or diabetes and cardiovascular risk factors like hypertension, dyslipidemia.

- Screening patients with leg-pain symptoms with exertion or abnormal lower extremity pulses.
- Screening people ≥ 70 years.
- Early diagnosis of lower-limb PAD using Ankle Brachial Pressure Index measurement. ABPI is considered sufficiently accurate so that verifying the diagnosis using arterial angiography is usually not recommended.
- Using the Edinburgh Claudication Questionnaire with the risk assessment.[2,3]
- Providing cardiovascular risk assessment and monitoring/follow-up, thus reducing risk of a serious cardiovascular event.
- Managing/alleviating current symptoms (pain, mobility).
- Aggresively treating risk factors and preventing events related to cardiovascular disease, disease progression and incapacity.
- Reducing hospital admission rate, invasive therapy (angioplasty, stenting) or surgery (amputation).
- Improving the patient's quality of life in the longer term and that of their family/carers.
- Sharing good practice, learning and skills with other providers in the local health community.
- Providing funding towards equipment (handheld Doppler with 8 MHz probe), nurse training and general practitioner time by the primary care trust.
- Making sure that clear protocols and patient pathways are in place for secondary care referral and further management if indicated.
- Providing service from a suitable general practice premises or community health clinic.
- Demonstrating a year-on-year improvement using the Quality and Outcomes Framework indicators – 40% improvement in achievement for cholesterol, hypertension and diabetes in year one, increasing to 60% in the second year and 80% in the third year.
- Complying with national requirements for recording, reporting, investigation and implementation of learning from incidents (National Patient Safety Agency).[4]

KEY POINTS

- The service framework aims to deliver a high-quality service in primary care for PAD patients.
- Primary care trusts need to consider addressing PAD in terms of case finding, provider capacity and informing local people earlier rather than later.

References

1 Vascular Society of Great Britain and Ireland. *The Provision of Services for Patients with Vascular Disease: 2009.* Available at: www.vascularsociety.org.uk/library/vascular-society-publications/doc_download/65-revised-provision-of-vascular-services-2004.html (accessed 10 March 2011).

2 Leng G, Fowkes F. The Edinburgh Claudication Questionnaire: an improved version of the WHO/Rose Questionnaire for use in epidemiological surveys. *J Clin Epidemiol.* 1992; **45**(10): 1101–9.

3 Fowkes FG, Housley E, Cawood EH *et al.* Edinburgh Artery Study: prevalence of asymptomatic and symptomatic peripheral arterial disease in the general population. *Int J Epidemiol.* 1991; **20**(2): 384–92.

4 www.npsa.nhs.uk (accessed 10 March 2011).

14

Secondary care referral

All patients with peripheral vascular disease (PVD) merit proper assessment. Most patients with intermittent claudication present at between 55 and 60 years of age. In most cases a conservative approach is all that is required, and this can be effectively delivered by a primary care physician. A primary care team can easily provide control of blood pressure, antiplatelet therapy, diabetic control and advice on stopping smoking and increasing exercise.

The heart protection study showed the benefits of simvastatin in a dose of 40 mg daily for patients with peripheral arterial disease. It improved the symptoms of PVD and also reduced the coronary events by 20%.[1,2] Again, this can be done in a primary care setting by a general practitioner.

The natural history of PVD is that a small percentage will deteriorate.

Data from the UK Office for National Statistics indicate that the number of people aged 60 years and over will rise from 12 million in 2001 to 18.6 million in 2031. The number of people with chronic disease and disability will also increase, and that increase will be threefold.[3] This will reflect the increasing need of vascular emergency units and specialists.

Atherosclerosis is more common in old age. With an increasing older population the number of atherosclerotic claudicants will also increase. It is well known that atherosclerotic claudication may cause myocardial infarction, transient ischaemic attack, stroke and possible loss of a limb, requiring hospital admission or surgical intervention. The overall 5-year mortality due to cardiovascular events including myocardial infarction is 20%–30%.[4] It is easy to dismiss this condition in a younger age group where atherosclerosis can cause a fatal outcome.

No one patient is the same. Different levels of understanding, compliance and concomitant disease all affect the suitability of treatment. Common sense dictates that each patient should be carefully examined, treated and referred to secondary care, if indicated, for early intervention to save a major amputation.

When to refer

Acute ischaemia of the leg

Acute ischaemia of the leg is most common among the older population. The outcome of this condition depends on the presence of comorbidities and the duration of ischaemia. Any patient with suspected or confirmed ischaemia must be admitted as an emergency case. This is essential if the limb is to be salvaged by reconstructive surgery. If the patient is treated within 24 hours the amputation rate is 9%, but after that the rate rises to 23%. For patients with severe ischaemia, peripheral arterial bypass surgery improves walking distance and quality of life significantly over other approaches.[5,6]

The classical symptoms of acute ischaemia are:[7]

- severe pain – the patient usually gets relief by hanging the leg over the edge of bed; however, pain may not be a feature in diabetics
- cold leg
- pallor
- absent pulses
- paraesthesia – diabetic patients may already have a sensory deficit that masks the change.

Remember 'Five Ps' for acute ischaemia:

Pale, Painful, Pulseless, Paraesthesia and Perishing (with cold).

Transient ischaemic attack

All patients with transient ischaemic attack (TIA) should be referred to the secondary care for examination of carotid arteries by a duplex scan. Patients with carotid stenosis > 70% benefit from carotid endarterectomy; however, death due to complications of ischaemic heart disease is the most common outcome in patients with TIA.[8]

Large multicentre trials show that surgery for high-grade carotid stenosis is beneficial in patients with symptoms of TIA.[9]

Suspected abdominal aneurysm

Most abdominal aneurysms are asymptomatic until rupture occurs. A detailed history and careful palpation of the abdomen, checking of the pulses, bruits and signs of peripheral ischaemia may give a clue and, if suspected, an urgent admission must be organised.

Rupture is estimated to have 85% mortality and causes 2% of deaths in men over the age of 65 years in United Kingdom;[10,11] ultrasound screening may be of value as it can detect an abdominal aortic aneurysm in 90% of cases.[10] It is estimated that the annual cost of a screening programme for abdominal aortic aneurysm in the United Kingdom would be less than £15 million, falling to £5 million within 10 years.[11]

Varicose vein

Referral to secondary care is necessary for relief of symptoms and prevention of complications. The most common reason for presentation to a general practitioner (GP) is cosmetic disfigurement, particularly in women. Endovenous obliteration using radiofrequency (diathermy) or laser, an alternative to the traditional stripping, or a minimally invasive procedure called powered phlebectomy are the current operative techniques for varicose veins. Trials have shown that both these techniques are acceptable alternative treatments.[12]

Bleeding from a varicosity that has eroded the skin or a varicosity that has bled and is at risk of another bleed warrants urgent referral to a vascular surgeon.

Deep-vein thrombosis

Pulmonary embolism is a serious complication of deep-vein thrombosis (DVT). All patients with a suspected DVT, bilateral DVT, Wells Risk Probability Score of 1 or more or patients who are pregnant should be referred to secondary care.

Vascular injury

Any suspicion of arterial injury following a road traffic accident attending a general practice surgery or asking for an appointment should be directed to the A&E/vascular unit (if available in the area) to prevent a fatal outcome.

Severe peripheral artery disease

Most patients with peripheral artery disease (PAD) will improve after a period of conservative management with an emphasis on reduction of risk factors. Referral to secondary care is indicated if claudication is significantly impairing the quality of life, if there is a severe case of PAD or if diagnosis is in doubt. Percutaneous balloon angioplasty has been shown to be effective in improving walking distance.

Ischaemic ulcer

Ischaemic ulcers can be caused by either progressive atherosclerosis or arterial embolisation. Both lead to ischaemia of the skin and ulceration. The common causes of ischaemic ulcers are diabetes mellitus, polyarteritis nodosa, rheumatoid arthritis, atherosclerosis and thromboangitis obliterans. Ischaemic ulcers are painful and patient reports pain especially at night relieved by dependency of the extremity. Provide adequate analgesia, help patient to stop smoking, address and control diabetes, blood pressure (remember beta blockers contraindicated), obesity and hyperlipidaemia and refer the patient to secondary care.

Neuropathic ulcer

Neuropathic ulcers are often seen underlying calluses or over pressure points (planter aspect of 1st or 5th metarsophalangeal joints). They are characterised by a punched out appearance with a deep sinus. These ulcers are painless because of neuropathy leading to hypesthesia. The neuropathic foot is warm, pink and has easily palpable pulses. The vibration, pinprick and light touch sensation are all reduced. Optimal control of blood sugar is very important. Neuropathic ulcers often take weeks to heal and the only way to ensure healing is to avoid weight bearing and an urgent referral.

Charcot's foot

Charcot's foot occurs most often in people with diabetes mellitus. It is a degenerative progressive condition that affects the joints in the feet. The joints affected are tarsal, metatarsal and tarsometatarsal. It is associated with neuropathy which decreases the ability to sense pain. As a result joints are subjected to repeated injury resulting in destruction of bones, ligaments and cartilage leading to severe deformity of the foot.

Raynaud's phenomenon

All symptomatic patients not responding to conservative treatment or severe cases presenting with digital ulceration or gangrene need an early assessment and management by the secondary care.

Lymphoedema causing chronic swelling of the leg

In a normal limb the hydrostatic pressure of the column of blood in the veins which depends on the integrity of the venous valves is balanced by the pump action of the calf muscle. The postphlebitic damage to valves, failure of the muscle pump, venous or lymphatic insufficiency, allergy, trauma or infection causing increased capillary permeability results in exudation of fluid rich in protein into the tissue spaces. Failure to remove protein because of lymphatic insufficiency results in oedema. It is not possible to cure lymphoedema. Majority patients benefit with raising the foot end of the bed and use of grade IV support stockings. It is important to maintain foot hygiene to avoid cellulitis. A few patients benefit from operations to relieve lymphatic obstruction.

Body mass index is more than 40 kg/m²

Refer for bariatric gastric surgery if body mass index (BMI) is more than $40 \, kg/m^2$. (Your primary care trust may have strict criteria of offering the procedure such as BMI of 50 or more.) Unfortunately, not a lot can be done if your referral gets rejected.

Peripheral arteriovenous malformation

Peripheral arteriovenous malformation is a rare presentation in general practice. Most are congenital lesions and are picked up at the time of birth and referral organised. Some appear years after birth because of either accidental or iatrogenic trauma and tend to be cosmetically unacceptable. (In my 22 years of general practice I have seen only two cases of port wine stain and one case of Sturge–Weber syndrome).

Others

Treatment failure, not sure about the diagnosis and severe refractory patients suffering with restless legs syndrome.

Useful websites

For patients

- Veins1 (www.veins1.com) for information on vein care for patients.
- Vascular Disease Foundation (www.vdf.org) for information on all aspects of vascular disease.

For GPs

- ScienceDirect (www.sciencedirect.com/science/journal/07415214) for information on vascular surgery.

KEY POINTS

- Refer to a vascular surgeon rather than a general surgeon. Outcomes for patients are better when arterial operations are done by a specialist.[13]
- The use of less invasive techniques for varicose vein surgery potentially lowers the risk of post-operative infection.

References

1 Burns P, Lima E, Bradbury AW. What constitutes best medical therapy for peripheral arterial disease? *Eur J Vasc Endovasc Surg.* 2002; **24**(1): 6–12.

2 Collins R, Peto R, Armitage J. The MRC/BHF heart protection study: preliminary results. *Int J Clin Pract.* 2002; **56**(1): 53–6.

3 Khaw KT. How many, how old, how soon? *BMJ.* 1999; **319**(7221): 1350–2.

4 Dormandy J, Heeck L, Vig S. The natural history of claudication: risk to life and limb. *Semin Vasc Surg.* 1999; **12**(2): 123–37.

5 Gelin J, Jivegard I, Taft C *et al.* Treatment efficacy of intermittent claudication by surgical intervention, supervised physical exercise training compared to no treatment in unselected randomised patients I: one year results of functional and physiological improvements. *Eur J Vasc Endovasc Surg.* 2001; **22**(2): 107–13.

6 Taft C, Karlsson J, Gelin J *et al.* Treatment efficacy of intermittent claudication by invasive therapy, supervised physical exercise training compared to no treatment in unselected randomised patients II: one-year results of health-related quality of life. *Eur J Vasc Endovasc Surg.* 2001; **22**(2): 114–23.

7 Wolfe JHN, (ed.) (2000) *ABC of Vascular Diseases.* London: *British Medical Journal.* pp. 15–18.

8 Hennessy MJ, Britton TC. Transient ischaemic attacks: evaluation and management. *Int J Clin Pract*. 2005; **54**(7): 432–6.

9 Rothwell PM, Gutnikov SA, Warlow CP. Reanalysis of the final results of the
European Carotid Surgery Trial. *Stroke*. 2003; **34**(2): 514–23.

10 Ashton HA, Buxton MJ, Day NE *et al*. The Multicentre Aneurysm Screening
Study (MASS) into the effect of abdominal aortic aneurysm screening on mortality in men: a randomised controlled trial. *Lancet*. 2002; **360**(9345): 1531–9.

11 Beard JD. Screening for abdominal aortic aneurysm. *Br J Surg*. 2003; **90**(5):
515–16.

12 Sybrandy JE, Wittens CH. Initial experiences in endovenous treatment of
saphenous vein reflux. *J Vasc Surg*. 2002; **36**(6): 1207–12.

13 Tu JV, Austin PC, Johnston KW. The influence of surgical specialty training
on the outcomes of elective abdominal aortic aneurysm surgery. *J Vasc Surg*.
2001; **33**(3): 447–52.

15

Commissioning services for peripheral vascular disease

Traditionally, GPs have always directed the flow of resources through a referral and prescribing activity. They are both providers (through their contract with primary care trust) and commissioners (through the referral of registered patients to secondary care or other providers). Practice based commissioning encourages GPs to make necessary referrals by adhering to 'care pathway protocols', to prescribe cost-effectively and to avoid unnecessary hospital follow-ups. Under practice-based commissioning, a primary care team can provide diagnostic services and preventive care thus reducing hospital admission. The boundary between the primary and secondary care interface is gradually being eroded as the care provided previously by the secondary care specialist is now provided by the primary care specialist in a primary care setting.

GPs have a major influence on what care a patient receives and how a patient can exercise choice.

The New Labour government gave birth to commissioning in the 1997. The previous 'purchasing' term used by conservative government was dropped and the culture of the 'competitive' market was replaced with 'collaboration' between purchasers (health authorities) and providers (hospitals, community services and mental health services).[1]

Commissioning can be interpreted in two entirely different ways. To some it means collaboration between primary care trusts and the GP practices and providers to determine the healthcare needs and how best to provide those in the most cost-effective way. To others, commissioning is the means geared to make primary care trusts a meaningful countervailing power to hospitals.[1]

When the Department of Health launched practice-based commissioning (PBC) in March 2005, most GPs were passionate about working together as commissioners. It promised whole scale improvements in the design and quality of service engaging all GPs.

In the beginning it had no clear agenda. Questions were raised. Was this about driving down referrals to help cash-strapped primary care trusts to balance their books or was this about enabling GPs to make money?

A recent Department of Health PBC quarterly survey revealed that only 68% of practices were even aware of being given an indicative budget, which is a fundamental prerequisite to commissioning. More than 30% of practices reported a 'poor' primary care trust support. This naturally demotivated GPs who made a conscious and considerate effort to commission services. Only 51% believed that PBC had improved patient care. We need to learn lessons from successful GP commissioners. These GPs became clinical leaders, shaping the service redesign. Competent primary care trust management with a high level of GP engagement was another reason for success.

There are many critics of PBC and with a change of government there could be changes to the scheme. According to one recently published report from the House of Commons Health Select Committee, the costs of commissioning are 14% of the real budget.[2] Two recent reports, produced jointly by the King's Fund and the Nuffield Trust,[3,4] suggest reviving the idea of GPs holding the purse strings for buying secondary care services. The Nuffield Trust and the King's Fund advocate 'integrated care' whereby primary and secondary care clinicians working together hold the real budgets and the primary care trusts operate as a separate higher-level commissioning organisation. For this to be successful the Nuffield report argues that primary care trusts will have to be larger, by merging with other trusts, to function as a separate high-level commissioning organisation.[3]

PBC needs to provide a quality primary care focusing on prevention and early management, using a community-based model. The aim is to prevent hospital admissions or patients turning up at A&E. This in itself will save a lot of money, which can be reinvested in patients' care.

The commissioning in peripheral vascular disease (PVD) can be achieved by identifying the objectives, providing cost-effective care of the highest possible quality and a good partnership arrangement with the primary care trust.

Why commission in PVD?

We are living in an era of patient choice, providing the best care to our patients under considerable economic constraints. The continual drive to improve the health of the population and economic viability has led to new shared care models of service delivery. Clinicians working together in a shared care offer the optimal management. The ongoing education of the primary care physician is equally important for the long-term sustainability of this model of care.

Intermittent claudication, a manifestation of PVD, is a common and debilitating condition that affects 1.7%–7.1% of people over the age of 55 years,[4] killing around 30% of patients within 5 years and 50% within 10 years because of cardiovascular disease,[5] with direct cost to the NHS of millions of pounds.

The truth is that patients with PVD are receiving suboptimal care in the United Kingdom. It deserves more attention and GPs can play a role in early identification and early management of this condition. Unfortunately, it is not a part of the Quality and Outcomes Framework – a reason why this is forgotten and neglected. Commissioning is the way forward.

Significant NHS savings can be made by commissioning services if patients are treated early with risk reduction therapies, preventing critical ischaemia resulting in amputation and reducing the unnecessary hospital referral. PBC is an effective tool to initiate clinical integration. Successful commissioning brings together primary care practitioners, hospital doctors and other service providers, including patients themselves.

The Royal College of General Practitioners and the Royal College of Physicians emphasise the importance of shared working as the most effective way of managing patients with chronic conditions.[6]

The major challenge for the NHS now is to combine quality with financial savings. This means shorter length of stay but with many more senior doctors per capita.[7] This can only work if commissioners and providers (doctors and hospitals) work together.

Why set up the service in primary healthcare?

- Better choice and flexibility for patients in line with the government's Patient Choice initiative.
- Freeing up hospital consultants' time to allow them to focus on more problematic patients.
- Enhancing the skills of GPs and the other primary care providers.

Planning

- Set up a multidisciplinary group. The group must have a secondary care specialist, a lead GP, practice nurse/trained vascular nurse, a representative from patient participation group and a primary care trust lead responsible for service delivery.
- Identify target group patients by computer search or repeat prescriptions, e.g. all smokers over the age of 45 years, diabetics, patients with metabolic syndrome or impaired fasting glycaemia, hypertensives, people with raised cholesterol > 5 mmol/L, low-density lipoprotein cholesterol (LDL-C) > 3 mmol/L, family history of premature cardiovascular disease (men aged under 55 years, women aged under 65 years), fasting triglycerides > 1.7 mmol/L, obese with a body mass index (BMI) of > 30 kg/m^2.
- Discuss the idea with a locality-based commissioning group and aim to deliver the service to their eligible patients – *free of charge*.
- Be innovative and offer your services further afield too.

Setting up

- Defining aims and objectives of the service provision.
- Early identification of intermittent claudication by taking a detailed history, general examination, cardiovascular evaluation paying particular attention to signs of peripheral ischaemia and checking the pulses. Early initiation of an appropriate treatment plan. Diabetes and hyperlipidaemia are the two major risk factors for peripheral arterial disease.[8,9] Early treatment is crucial.
- Making best use of resources.
- Using the Edinburgh Claudication Questionnaire for symptomatic patients to detect peripheral arterial disease.[10]

- Measuring Ankle Brachial Pressure Index by using a handheld Doppler to screen at-risk groups.
- Using a dedicated PVD template. The template must include history of smoking, weight, height, BMI, blood pressure, lipid profile, blood sugar and examination of peripheral pulses. At present there is no such template. A person with a bit of knowledge about the computer system can easily create a PVD template.
- Agreeing on goals of treatment, e.g. smoking cessation (www. smokefree.nhs.uk/resources), exercise therapy[11] and medical management – for example, which cost-effective statin[12] to use and at what dose defining and agreeing the target level to reach as per evidence-based medicine. However, if blood-pressure-lowering drugs are required, which ACE (angiotensin-converting enzyme) inhibitor to use. The HOPE (Heart Outcomes Prevention Evaluation) study showed that ramipril reduces cardiovascular morbidity and mortality in peripheral arterial disease by 25%.[13]
- Involving the medicine management team, especially the locality's prescribing lead of the primary care trust, aiming to stay within the prescribing budget.
- Agreeing on referral indicators to secondary care.

Clinical governance

- Making sure that all equipments meet the necessary quality control and assurance standards.
- Having regular monthly meetings to evaluate the running of the service and making changes if necessary to improve the service provision.
- Getting as much feedback as possible by using patient satisfaction questionnaires.
- Recording all significant events with learning points and complaints.
- Keeping a training log and making sure staff providing the service are competent.
- Doing an audit at the end of 6 months, with clear aims and objectives.

Why audit?

For healthcare professionals the ability to provide good-quality care and for that care to be valued by others is fundamental to their sense of commitment. By doing regular audits the health professionals become even more confident that they can meet all the requirements of the people they serve. An audit is about setting standards for your performance, finding out how you are doing it, making changes and then re-auditing it.

An audit can be a quantitative audit or a significant event audit. One example of a quantitative audit could be to monitor the management of cholesterol targets with cost-effective statin-simvastatin in PVD, or how many symptomatic/asymptomatic patients had a Doppler test done.

A significant event audit is if something significant happens – for example, a pregnant woman attends with a swollen leg, diagnosis of DVT is missed and she gets admitted with pulmonary embolism. This means time for reflection, studying the facts, analysing the weaknesses/deficits/errors and determining which action should follow.

Prescribing advisors and audit managers in the primary care trust can supply information about your prescribing and performance indicators that may be useful in carrying out an audit.

Commissioning process

1 Decide why to commission this service.
2 Evaluate the existing service.
3 Plan the service.
4 Implement.
5 Monitor (clinical governance).

National organisations

There are various national organisations that can provide help and support for PBC.

- National Association of Primary Care (www.napc.co.uk).
- Improvement Foundation (UK) http://Communityhealthsupport. org/2009/p_30.php.
- Department of Health. *The NHS in England: the operating framework for 2008/9* (www.dh.gov.uk/en/Publicationsandstatistics/Publications/ PublicationsPolicyAndGuidance/DH_081094 (accessed 10 March 2011)).

KEY POINTS

- Commissioning in PVD can deliver an earlier diagnosis and earlier initiation of an appropriate management plan to reduce the cardiovascular risk.
- Risk factors can be easily and effectively managed in the primary care setting by commissioning.
- Integrated care organisations are likely to become increasingly important for service delivery, according to the most recent Department of Health PBC guidance (March 2009).

References

1 Paton C. Commissioning in the English NHS. *BMJ*. 2010; **340**: c1979.

2 House of Commons – Health Committee Reports Fourth report. *Commissioning*. 30 March 2010. Available at: www.publications.parliament.uk/pa/cm200910/cmselect/cmhealth/268/26802.htm (accessed 10 March 2011).

3 Smith J, Curry N, Mays N *et al. Where Next for Commissioning in the English NHS?* London: Nuffield Trust; 15 April 2010. Available at: www.nuffieldtrust.org.uk/publications/detail.aspx?id=145&prID=694 (accessed 10 March 2011).

4 Fowkes F, Housley E, Cawood EH *et al.* Edinburgh Artery Study: prevalence of asymptomatic and symptomatic peripheral arterial disease in the general population. *Int J Epidemiol*. 1991; **20**(2): 384–92.

5 Atwal A. Intermittent claudication. 2000. www.highbeam.com/doc/1G1-106648568.html (accessed 10 March 2011).

6 Royal College of Physicians of London, Royal College of General Practitioners, NHS Alliance. *Clinicians, Services and Commissioning in Chronic Disease Management in the NHS: the need for coordinated management programmes*. London: Royal College of Physicians of London; 2004.

7 Feachem RGA, Sekhri NK, White KL *et al.* Getting more for their dollar: a comparison of the NHS with California's Kaiser Permanente. *BMJ*. 2002; **324**(7330): 135–41.

8 American Diabetes Association. Peripheral arterial disease in people with diabetes. *Diabetes Care*. 2003; **26**(12): 3333–41.

9 Jude E, Gibbons J. Identifying and treating intermittent claudication in people with diabetes. *Diabetic Foot Journal*. 2005; **8**(2): 84–92.

10 Leng GC, Fowkes FG. The Edinburgh Claudication Questionnaire. *J Clin Epidemiol.* 1992; **45**(10): 1101–9.

11 Leng GC, Fowler B, Ernst E. Exercise for intermittent claudication (Cochrane Review). In: *The Cochrane Library.* Issue 2. Chichester: John Wiley & Sons; 2000.

12 Heart Protection Study Collaborative Group. MRC/BHF Heart protection study of cholesterol lowering with simvastatin in 20,536 high-risk individuals: a randomised placebo-controlled trial. *Lancet.* 2002; **360**(9326): 7–22.

13 Yusuf S, Sleight P, Pogue J *et al.* Effects of an angiotensin-converting-enzyme inhibitor, ramipril, on cardiovascular events in high-risk patients. The Heart Outcomes Prevention Evaluation Study Investigators. *N Engl J Med.* 2000; **342**(3): 145–53.

16

One-stop clinic

Chronic disease takes up a massive part of the National Health Service's (NHS) resources and its management is actually the future of the NHS. Patients with chronic conditions are more likely to see their general practitioner (GP). The aim is to develop new ways of thinking about chronic disease management.

The Royal College of Physicians, the Royal College of General Practitioners and the NHS Alliance published the results of a joint working party in a report entitled *Clinicians, Services and Commissioning in Chronic Disease Management in the NHS*, emphasising the need for the coordinated programme in managing the chronic disease.[1] The document focuses on the clinician-led service change, joint approaches at a local level setting up clinical directorates that span primary and secondary care, joint working, information sharing, greater leadership training for the clinicians and the development of training programmes. This brought new challenges and opportunities for those GPs who were keen to expand their roles in the speciality of their choice.

The management of peripheral vascular disease (PVD) in a primary care setting is an obvious choice for those GPs with a real enthusiasm and interest in vascular disease. These specialist GPs can provide local, high-quality and timely management to patients with vascular problems by providing a one-stop clinic in the primary care setting.

The Quality and Outcomes Framework (QOF) awarded 257 clinical points out of 550 for the management of coronary heart disease in the original QOF because cardiovascular disease causes 37% of premature deaths in males and 27% in females. Peripheral arterial disease (PAD) is one of the biggest risk factors for coronary heart disease. Forty-three per cent of patients with claudication symptoms develop coronary heart disease, 24% will have heart failure and 21% will have a stroke within 10 years.[2]

The QOF awarded practices with incentives to bring down cholesterol levels, target blood pressure as per guidelines and address HbA1c level in diabetic control; however, it offered nothing for vascular checks. Some clinicians thought that this omission from the original Quality and Outcomes Framework was illogical.[3] It was hoped that PAD would be included in the first review of Quality and Outcomes Framework for GMS contract; however, it was ignored again.

A one-stop clinic in a primary care setting can provide the following.

- Diagnosis of the lower-limb PVD using Ankle Brachial Pressure Index (ABPI) measurement.
- Cardiovascular disease (CVD) risk assessment, prevention, monitoring and follow-up.
- Management of risk factors (cholesterol, blood pressure, weight, smoking cessation); Target PAD (www.targetpad.co.uk) is a group focusing on raising awareness of PAD so that patients can benefit from earlier treatment and therefore a reduction in the number of cardiovascular events.
- Weight management. If the patient needs help regarding weight, eating less and exercising more is sometimes not good enough: empathy and care can be shown by helping them into a weight management programme. Drugs like orlistat can be prescribed if body mass index (BMI) > 28 kg/m^2 and other comorbidities are present. NICE (National Institute for Health and Clinical Excellence) guidelines suggest referral for bariatric gastric surgery if BMI > 40 kg/m^2 or 35 kg/m^2 with comorbidities.[4,5]
- Advice on waist circumference – ideally it should be < 102 cm in men (< 92 cm for Asian men) and < 88 cm in women (< 78 cm for Asian women).
- Management and maintenance of target lipid levels by selecting an appropriate cost-effective statin.
- Improvement of compliance to treatment.
- Review of the treatment, and monitoring of side effects or drug interactions.

- Symptom management, improving walking distance by encouraging exercise, providing exercise on prescription if available in the area.
- Reduction of disease progression by organising regular follow-ups.
- Organisation of early referral to vascular surgeon for further investigation if ABPI > 1.3.
- Sharing of good practice.
- Teaching and training.
- Reduction of the secondary care specialist's workload, allowing them to concentrate on difficult patients.
- Provision of in-house surgery by deploying new techniques of endovascular laser, ultrasound and foam therapy, now a popular choice for varicose vein surgery. This can easily be done in a primary care setting.
- Providing echocardiogram,[6] carotid artery scanning[7] in a primary care setting for assessment of vascular risk factors.

Quality indicators specific to cholesterol management: GMS contract[8]

TABLE 16.1 Cholesterol: Indicators, points and payment stages

INDICATOR	POINTS	PAYMENT STAGES
Ongoing management		
CHD 7. The percentage of patients with coronary heart disease whose notes have a record of total cholesterol in the previous 15 months	7	40%–90%
CHD 8. The percentage of patients with coronary heart disease whose last measured total cholesterol (measured in previous 15 months) is 5 mmol/L or less	17	40%–70%
Stroke 7. The percentage of patients with TIA or stroke who have a record of total cholesterol in the last 15 months	2	40%–90%
Stroke 8. The percentage of patients with TIA or stroke whose last measured total cholesterol (measured in the previous 15 months) is 5 mmol/L or less	5	40%–60%

(continued)

INDICATOR	POINTS	PAYMENT STAGES
DM 16. The percentage of patients with diabetes who have a record of total cholesterol in the previous 15 months	3	40%–90%
DM 17. The percentage of patients with diabetes whose last measured total cholesterol within the previous 15 months is 5 mmol/L or less	6	40%–70%

Source: Adapted from the Quality and Outcomes Framework 2009/10 Guidance for GMS Contract[8]

Targets recommended by JBS 2[9]

- Total cholesterol < 4 mmol/L or 25% reduction, whichever is lower.
- Low-density lipoprotein cholesterol (LDL-C) < 2 mmol/L or 30% reduction, whichever is lower.

Quality indicators specific to blood pressure: GMS contract[8]

TABLE 16.2 Blood pressure: Indicators, points and payment stages

INDICATOR	POINTS	PAYMENT STAGES
Ongoing management		
The percentage of patients with hypertension in whom there is a record of the blood pressure in the previous 9 months	18	40%–90%
The percentage of patients with hypertension in whom the last blood pressure (measured in the previous 9 months) is 150/90 or less	57	40%–70%

Source: Adapted from the Quality and Outcomes Framework 2009/10 Guidance for GMS Contract[8]

Blood pressure (BP) readings taken in the surgery can sometimes provide an inaccurate measurement if a patient appears nervous or stressed. In these situations self-monitoring of BP should be encouraged. The cost of good, reliable self-monitoring devices is roughly under £50. The British Hypertension Society encourages the self-monitoring of BP. Encourage the patient to buy a self-monitoring device or the clinic can loan one.

Target blood pressure

TABLE 16.3 Target blood pressure

TRIAL	PATIENT POPULATION	TARGET BP
HOT (Hypertension optimal treatment)	Hypertension	Diastolic < 80
ALLHAT (Antihypertensive and lipid lowering treatment to prevent heart attack trial)	Hypertension plus at least one other CVD risk factor	< 140/90
ASCOT (Anglo-Scandinavian Cardiac Outcome Trial – blood pressure lowering arm)	Hypertension plus at least three other CVD risk factors	< 140/90 < 130/80 with diabetes

Further reading

Self-help guides for patients

- Diabetes UK www.diabetes.org.uk.

Healthy eating and exercise

- British Heart Foundation (www.bhf.org.uk).
- Eatwell (www.eatwell.gov.uk).

Stopping smoking

- Clinical Knowledge Summaries (www.cks.library.nhs.uk).
- Giving up smoking www.quit.org.uk.
- NHS smoking helpline 0800 022 4332.
- Gosmokefree (www.gosmokefree.co.uk).
- Smoking/Patient UK. National Institute for Health and Clinical Excellence (NICE) (www.patient.co.uk.).

Self-monitoring BP

- British Hypertension Society – for information on BP monitors (www.bhsoc. org/blood_pressure_list.stm).
- British Hypertension Society – for information on BP measurement techniques (www.bhsoc.org/how_to_measure_blood_pressure.stm).

Useful reference for GPs

- NHS Evidence-Vascular provides evidence-based information on all aspects of vascular care. (www.library.nhs.uk) >Specialist Collections > Vascular Home.

KEY POINTS

- A one-stop clinic can provide local, timely and high-quality care to patients with PAD.
- Primary care is well placed to meet the challenge of cholesterol targets.
- Evidence suggests that patients could benefit from taking weight-reducing drugs like orlistat. The treatment should continue even after the weight plateaus to reduce possible weight gain.
- The stimulus of the new General Medical Services contract is encouraging GPs to facilitate the care needed to support the delivery of the good quality care.
- Endovenous laser and foam therapy can be performed in treatment rooms rather than operating theatres.

References

1 Royal College of Physicians of London, Royal College of General Practitioners, NHS Alliance. *Clinicians, Services and Commissioning in Chronic Disease Management in the NHS: the need for coordinated management programmes.* London: Royal College of Physicians of London; 2004.

2 Kennel WB. The demographics of claudication and the aging of the American population. *Vasc Med.* 1996; **1**(1): 60–4.

3 Jarvis S. The new GMS contract QOF update. *Br J Cardiol.* 2005; **12**(6): 413–15.

4 National Institute for Health and Clinical Excellence. *Obesity: the prevention, identification, assessment and management of overweight and obesity in adults and children: NICE guideline 43.* London: NIHCE; 2006. www.nice.org.uk/cg43.

5 www.nationalobesityforum.org.uk.

6 Savill P. GPwSI in cardiology: a personal view. *Clin Foc Prim Care.* 2005; **1**(1): 25–7.

7 Warlow CP, Davenport RJ. The management of transient ischaemic attacks. *Prescribers' Journal.* 1996; **36**(1): 1–8.

8 British Medical Association, NHS Employers. *Revisions to the GMS Contract*

2006/7: delivering investment in general practice [Quality and Outcomes Framework guidance]. 23 Feb 2006. Available at: www.nhsemployer.org/gmscontract.

9 British Cardiac Society, British Hypertension Society, Diabetes UK *et al.* JBS 2: Joint British Societies' guidelines on prevention of cardiovascular disease in clinical practice. *Heart.* 2005; **91**(5): v1–52.

17

Multiple-choice questions

1 An intravenous drug misuser with a deep-vein thrombosis (DVT) should be treated with:
   a) warfarin
   b) unfractionated heparin
   c) low-molecular-weight heparin
   d) a combination of warfarin and heparin
   e) nothing – leave alone.

2 The optimum duration of anticoagulation for a DVT for patients after the first thrombosis with no risk factors is:
   a) 6 weeks
   b) 10 weeks
   c) 12 weeks
   d) 3–6 months
   e) 6 months.

3 The optimum duration of anticoagulation for recurrent pulmonary embolism is:
   a) 3 weeks
   b) 3 months
   c) 10 weeks
   d) 12 months
   e) lifelong.

4 To prevent DVT, patients on long-haul flights should be advised to:
   a) drink tea and coffee
   b) drink gin and tonic
   c) take aspirin
   d) drink plenty of water to prevent dehydration
   e) walk around and regularly flex the ankles.

5 An Ankle Brachial Pressure Index (ABPI) measurement diagnostic of peripheral arterial disease (PAD) is:
   a) < 0.9
   b) > 0.9
   c) $= 0.9$
   d) < 0.3
   e) 2.0.

6 Symptom diagnostic of vascular claudication is:
   a) pain at rest
   b) pain that occurs in the calf muscles on walking and resolves with rest
   c) weakness of legs
   d) numbness of legs
   e) tiredness.

7 The first-line drug therapy for intermittent claudication is:
   a) naftidrofuryl
   b) nifedipine
   c) prednisolone
   d) cilostazol
   e) iron.

8 The only absolute contraindication of measuring ABPI is:
   a) DVT recently or within 6 weeks
   b) hypertensive patient
   c) poorly controlled diabetic
   d) history of claudication
   e) Raynaud's phenomenon.

9   The most common site of claudication pain is the:
   a) arm
   b) face
   c) calf
   d) chest
   e) head.

10   Severity of claudication is determined by:
   a) the World Health Organisation (WHO) classification
   b) the Heart Outcomes Prevention Evaluation (HOPE) classification
   c) the Intermittent Claudication Society
   d) Fontaine classification
   e) none of the above.

11   Critical ischaemia means:
   a) intermittent claudication
   b) no symptoms
   c) rest pain
   d) tingling
   e) tissue loss.

12   Patients with intermittent claudication should:
   a) rest
   b) exercise
   c) continue to smoke
   d) take calcium and vitamin D
   e) take omega-3 capsules.

13   The treatment of choice for high blood pressure (BP) in a patient with
     peripheral vascular disease (PVD) should be:
   a) thiazide diuretic
   b) beta blocker
   c) nifedipine
   d) ACE (angiotensin-converting enzyme) inhibitor
   e) furosemide.

14 Patients with PAD should be on:
   a) dipyridamole
   b) clopidogrel
   c) a combination of clopidogrel and dipyridamole
   d) aspirin unless contraindication
   e) none of the above.

15 Pain related to varicose veins is:
   a) worse in the morning
   b) worse when lying down
   c) worse towards the end of the day
   d) worse after elevating the leg
   e) worse after being seated for a period of time.

16 The following is true in restless legs syndrome (RLS):
   a) it has an estimated prevalence of 50%–60%
   b) beta blockers in low dose are helpful
   c) all patients should be treated with drug therapy
   d) dopamine agonists are the mainstay of treatment
   e) patients should avoid exercise.

17 RLS can be associated with deficiency of:
   a) vitamin C
   b) vitamin B_{12}
   c) iron
   d) calcium
   e) folate.

18 CHADS2 is a risk assessment tool used for:
   a) commencing warfarin
   b) initiating drug treatment in RLS
   c) assessing which patients with varicose veins should have surgery
   d) before initiating aspirin
   e) PVD.

19 Thromboembolic risk is increased in patients treated with warfarin if international normalised ratio (INR) is:
a) < 2
b) < 3
c) > 4
d) > 5
e) between 2 and 3.

20 The new, updated guidelines suggest aiming at an HbA1c target of:
a) 7%
b) 7.5%
c) 6.5%
d) 6%
e) 8%.

21 Lipid targets for type 2 diabetics are:
a) total cholesterol less than 4 mmol/Litre
b) total cholesterol less than 5 mmol/Litre
c) low-density lipoprotein cholesterol (LDL-C) of 3.0 mmol/Litre
d) high-density lipoprotein cholesterol (HDL-C) less than 3 mmol/Litre
e) total cholesterol less than 4 mmol/Litre and LDL-C of less than 2.0 mmol/Litre.

22 The following is true about compression stockings:
a) full-length stockings are better than below-knee stockings
b) class 2 is better than class 1
c) stockings should be avoided if the ABPI measurement is less than 0.9
d) stockings prevent the progression and recurrence after surgery of DVT
e) stockings are no longer prescribable.

23 The following are all common predisposing factors for development of varicose veins except:
a) obesity
b) previous DVT
c) parity in women

    d) prolonged standing

    e) male gender.

24 The risk of thrombosis is higher in all except:
    a) progestogen-only pills (POP)
    b) combined oral contraceptive pills (COC)
    c) those with body mass index (BMI) > 30
    d) carrier of hereditary thrombotic conditions
    e) smokers.

25 The only absolute contraindications for combined oral contraceptive pills (COC) are:
    a) wheelchair-bound
    b) BMI 30–39
    c) BMI > 39
    d) varicose veins
    e) normal clotting factors.

26 The following is true:
    a) oestrogens increase the high-density lipoprotein cholesterol (HDL-cholesterol)
    b) progestogens increase the high-density lipoprotein cholesterol (HDL-cholesterol)
    c) oestrogens reduce the blood pressure
    d) oestrogens increase the antithrombin 111 level
    e) oestrogens reduce the hepatic secretions of plasma proteins.

27 The Quality and Outcomes Framework target blood pressure is:
    a) 150/90
    b) same as the National Institute for Health and Clinical Excellence/British Hypertension Society target
    c) 140/85
    d) 150/100
    e) 145/85.

28 Resistant hypertension is defined as:
    a) uncontrolled hypertension

b) uncontrolled with treatment

c) patient resistant to taking treatment

d) uncontrolled despite treatment with optimum doses of at least three antihypertensive drugs

e) uncontrolled with maximum dose of beta blocker.

29 The first-line treatment for painful diabetic neuropathy, as per NICE guidelines, is:

a) morphine

b) oxycodone

c) tramadol

d) pregabalin

e) duloxetine.

30 The signs and symptoms of ischaemic foot are:

a) warm to touch

b) knee/ankle jerk diminished or absent

c) normal or pink colour

d) pale or cyanosed colour

e) diminished/absent sensation.

31 The signs and symptoms of neuropathic foot are:

a) warm to touch

b) diminished or absent sensations

c) absent or diminished dorsalis pedis

d) knee/ankle jerk present

e) cyanosed colour.

32 Refer to specialised foot care team if:

a) new ulceration

b) discolouration

c) poor vision/house bound

d) normal pulsation

e) normal sensation.

33 Hyperalgesia is:

a) no response following a pinprick

b) slight pain following pinprick

c) increased feeling of hot

d) increased sweating

e) exaggerated response to a pinprick.

34 Neuropathic pain is common in:
   a) herpes simplex
   b) men
   c) osteoarthritis of spine
   d) diabetes mellitus
   e) herpes zoster.

35 The drug commonly used for intermittent claudication is:
   a) paracetamol
   b) codeine
   c) cilostazol
   d) simvastatin
   e) morphine.

36 The commonest cause of secondary RLS is:
   a) iron deficiency anaemia
   b) diabetes
   c) renal failure
   d) vitamin C deficiency
   e) hypothyroid.

37 Drugs that may aggravate RLS are:
   a) beta blockers
   b) lithium
   c) Selective serotonin reuptake inhibitors (SSRI)
   d) ACE inhibitors
   e) nifedipine.

38 The mainstay of treatment of RLS is:
   a) folic acid
   b) beta blockers
   c) amlodipine

d) hypnotics

e) dopamine agonist.

39 Malignant hypertension is:
a) BP 180/110
b) BP 190/100
c) BP 200/100
d) BP 190/110
e) BP 190/110.

40 Red-flag symptoms in hypertension include:
a) papilloedema
b) fits
c) BP 180/110
d) headaches
e) signs of end-organ damage.

41 Target INR for DVT is:
a) 1.0
b) 2.0
c) 2.5
d) 6.0
e) 6.5.

42 Target INR for recurrence of venous thromboembolism while on warfarin is:
a) 1.0
b) 2.0
c) 2.5
d) 3.5
e) 4.5.

43 The following is a true statement about heparin:
a) heparin is given orally
b) heparin's half-life is 2 hours
c) heparin's half-life is 2 days
d) heparin is given subcutaneously

e) heparin works by inhibiting vitamin K-dependent factors.

44 Major risk factors for venous thromboembolism are:
a) major abdominal/pelvic surgery
b) varicose veins
c) hypertension
d) cardiac failure
e) malignancy.

45 Cause for a raised INR is:
a) heavy smoking
b) binge alcohol consumption
c) incorrect dose of warfarin
d) broad-spectrum antibiotics
e) rifampicin.

Answers

1 c
2 a
3 e
4 e
5 a
6 b
7 d
8 a
9 c
10 d
11 c and e
12 b
13 d
14 d
15 c*
16 d
17 c

---

* Pain related to varicose veins is worse after prolonged standing, or towards the end of the day, and is relieved by leg elevation.

18   a
19   a
20   c
21   e
22   c
23   e
24   a
25   c
26   a
27   a
28   d
29   e
30   d
31   a and b
32   a, b and c
33   e
34   d and e
35   c
36   a
37   a, b and c
38   e
39   a
40   a, b, c, d and e
41   c
42   d
43   b and d
44   a, b and e
45   b, c and d

Index